TABLE OF CONTENTS

Top 20 Test Taking Tips

1. Carefully follow all the test registration procedures
2. Know the test directions, duration, topics, question types, how many questions
3. Setup a flexible study schedule at least 3-4 weeks before test day
4. Study during the time of day you are most alert, relaxed, and stress free
5. Maximize your learning style; visual learner use visual study aids, auditory learner use auditory study aids
6. Focus on your weakest knowledge base
7. Find a study partner to review with and help clarify questions
8. Practice, practice, practice
9. Get a good night's sleep; don't try to cram the night before the test
10. Eat a well balanced meal
11. Know the exact physical location of the testing site; drive the route to the site prior to test day
12. Bring a set of ear plugs; the testing center could be noisy
13. Wear comfortable, loose fitting, layered clothing to the testing center; prepare for it to be either cold or hot during the test
14. Bring at least 2 current forms of ID to the testing center
15. Arrive to the test early; be prepared to wait and be patient
16. Eliminate the obviously wrong answer choices, then guess the first remaining choice
17. Pace yourself; don't rush, but keep working and move on if you get stuck
18. Maintain a positive attitude even if the test is going poorly
19. Keep your first answer unless you are positive it is wrong
20. Check your work, don't make a careless mistake

Foundations of Advanced Nursing Practice

Cerebral aneurysms

Cerebral aneurysms, weakening and dilation of a cerebral artery, are usually congenital (90%) while the remaining (10%) result from direct trauma or infection. Aneurysms usually range from 2-7 mm and occur in the Circle of Willis at the base of the brain. A rupturing aneurysm may decrease perfusion as well as increasing pressure on surrounding brain tissue, resulting in mental changes. Cerebral aneurysms are classified as follows:

- Berry/saccular: The most common congenital type occurs at a bifurcation and grows from the base on a stem, usually at the Circle of Willis.
- Fusiform: Large and irregular (>2.5 cm) and rarely ruptures, but causes increased intracranial pressure. Usually involves the internal carotid or vertebrobasilar artery.
- Mycotic: Rare type that occurs secondary to bacterial infection and a septic emboli.
- Dissecting: Wall is torn apart and blood enters layers. This may occur during angiography or secondary to trauma or disease.
- Traumatic Charcot-Bouchard (pseudoaneurysm): Small lesion resulting from chronic hypertension.

Astrocytoma, brain stem glioma, craniopharyngioma, and meningioma

Any type of brain tumor can occur in children and adults. Brain tumors may cause psychiatric symptoms, such as hallucinations and changes in mental status, depending on the type and site. Brain tumors are classified as follows:

- Astrocytoma: Arises from astrocytes, which are glial cells. It is the most common type of tumor, occurring throughout the brain but most common in the cerebellum of children. There are many types of astrocytomas, and most are slow growing. Some are operable while others are not. Radiation may be given after removal. Astrocytomas include glioblastomas, aggressively malignant tumors occurring most often in adults 45-70.
- Brain stem glioma: May be fast or slow growing but generally not operable because of location, although it may be treated with radiation or chemotherapy.
- Craniopharyngioma: A congenital, slow-growing, and benign cystic tumor; however, it is difficult to resect and is treated with surgery and radiation. May be recurrent, especially if >5 cm.
- Meningioma: Slow-growing meningeal tumor, usually benign and more common in women; surgically removed if causing symptoms.

Arteriovenous malformation

Arteriovenous malformation (AVM) is a congenital abnormality characterized by a tangle of dilated arteries and veins without a capillary bed. AVMs can occur anywhere in the brain and may cause no significant problems. Usually the AVM is "fed" by 1 or more cerebral arteries, which enlarge over time, shunting more blood through the AVM. The veins also enlarge in response to increased arterial blood flow because of the lack of a capillary bridge between the 2. Because vein walls are thinner and lack the muscle layer of an artery, the veins tend to rupture as the AVM becomes larger, causing a subarachnoid hemorrhage. Chronic ischemia that may be related to the AVM can result in cerebral atrophy. Sometimes small leaks, usually accompanied by headache, nausea, and vomiting,

may occur before rupture. AVMs may cause a wide range of neurological symptoms, including changes in mentation, dizziness, sensory abnormalities, confusion, and dementia. Treatment includes:
- Supportive management of symptoms.
- Surgical repair or focused irradiation (definitive treatments).

Strokes

Strokes (brain attacks, cerebrovascular accidents) result when there is interruption of the blood flow to an area of the brain. The 2 basic types are ischemic and hemorrhagic. About 80% are ischemic, resulting from blockage of an artery supplying the brain. Ischemic strokes are classified as follows:
- Thrombosis in large artery, usually resulting from atherosclerosis, may block circulation to a large area of the brain. It is most common in the elderly and may occur suddenly or after episodes of transient ischemic attacks.
- Lacunar infarct (penetrating thrombosis in small artery) is most common in those with diabetes mellitus and/or hypertension.
- Embolism travels through the arterial system and lodges in the brain, most commonly in the left middle cerebral artery. An embolism may be cardiogenic, resulting from cardiac arrhythmia or surgery. An embolism usually occurs rapidly with no warning signs.
- Cryptogenic has no identifiable cause.

Hemorrhagic strokes account for about 20% of all strokes and result from a ruptured cerebral artery, causing not only lack of oxygen and nutrients but also edema that causes widespread pressure and damage. Hemorrhagic strokes are classified as follows:
- Intracerebral is bleeding into the substance of the brain from an artery in the central lobes, basal ganglia, pons, or cerebellum. Intracerebral hemorrhage usually results from atherosclerotic degenerative changes, hypertension, brain tumors, anticoagulation therapy, or some illicit drugs, such as crack and cocaine. Onset is often sudden and may cause death.
- Intracranial aneurysm occurs with ballooning cerebral artery ruptures, most commonly at the Circle of Willis.
- Arteriovenous malformation (AVM) is a tangle of dilated arteries and veins without a capillary bed. This is a congenital abnormality. Rupture of AVMs is a cause of stroke in young adults.
- Subarachnoid hemorrhage is bleeding in the space between the meninges and brain, resulting from aneurysm, AVM, or trauma. This type of hemorrhage compresses brain tissue.

Strokes most commonly occur in the right or left hemisphere, but the exact location and the extent of brain damage affects the type of presenting symptoms. If the frontal area of either side is involved, there tends to be memory and learning deficits. Some symptoms are common to specific areas and help to identify the area involved:
- Right hemisphere: This results in left paralysis or paresis and a left visual field deficit that may cause spatial and perceptual disturbances so that people may have difficulty judging distance. Fine motor skills may be impacted, resulting in trouble dressing or handling tools. People may become impulsive and exhibit poor judgment, often denying impairment. Left-sided neglect (lack of perception of things on the left side) may occur. Depression is common as well as short-term memory loss and difficulty following directions. Language skills usually remain intact.

- Left hemisphere: This results in right paralysis or paresis and a right visual field defect. Depression is common and people often exhibit slow, cautious behavior, requiring repeated instruction and reinforcement for simple tasks. Short-term memory loss and difficulty learning new material or understanding generalizations is common. Difficulty with mathematics, reading, writing, and reasoning may occur. Aphasia (expressive, receptive, or global) is common.
- Brain stem: Because the brain stem controls respiration and cardiac function, a brain attack frequently causes death, but those who survive may have a number of problems, including respiratory and cardiac abnormalities. Strokes may involve motor or sensory impairment or both.
- Cerebellum: This area controls balance and coordination. Strokes in the cerebellum are rare but may result in ataxia, nausea, and vomiting, as well as headaches and dizziness or vertigo.

Hydrocephalus

Hydrocephalus occurs when there is an imbalance between production and absorption of cerebrospinal fluid (CSF) in the ventricles, resulting from impaired absorption or obstruction, which may be congenital or acquired. The ventricular system produces and circulates CSF. There are right and left lateral ventricles, which open into the third ventricle at the interventricular foramen (foramen of Monro). The aqueduct of Sylvius connects the third and fourth ventricles. The fourth ventricle, anterior to the cerebellum, supplies CSF to the subarachnoid space and the spinal cord (dorsal surface). The CSF circulates and then returns to the brain and is absorbed in the arachnoid villi. There are 2 common types of hydrocephalus:

- Communicating: CSF flows (communicates) between the ventricles but is not absorbed in the subarachnoid space (arachnoid villi).
- Non-communicating: CSF is obstructed (non-communicating) between the ventricles with obstruction, often resulting in stenosis of the aqueduct of Sylvius, but it can occur anywhere in the system.

Multiple sclerosis

Multiple sclerosis (MS) is a central nervous system (CNS) immune-mediated inflammatory demyelinating disease, believed triggered by an unidentified environmental source, such as a virus. MS is associated with mood swings, depression, and changes in mental status. Within the CNS, small glial cells, oligodendrocytes, send out processes that wrap around the axons of neurons, creating the myelin sheath. One oligodendrocyte may "grasp" 10-15 neurons, and adjoining segments of the sheath are created by other oligodendrocytes, with spaces in between (Nodes of Ranvier). The sheath, primarily composed of lipids, is white in appearance, creating the "white matter" of the brain. Impulses travel along the sheath, jumping from 1 node to another. With MS, for reasons that are not clear, an immune reaction causes killer T cells to attack the oligodendrocytes, which begin to demyelinate, leaving scarred areas along the axons, slowing neuronal transmission. Damage to 1 oligodendrocyte can affect many neurons. Initially, unaffected mature oligodendrocytes repair the damage, so symptoms tend to wax and wane. Over time, however, cells cannot remyelinate and new cells don't develop adequately, so symptoms worsen.

Parkinson's disease

Parkinson's disease (PD) is an extrapyramidal movement motor system disorder caused by loss of brain cells that produce dopamine. The basal ganglia, which lies at the base of the cerebral cortex and controls movement and coordination, has a number of structures that are involved in PD, particularly the substantia nigra, where neuronal cells project fibers to the putamen and caudate of the corpus striatum, releasing dopamine (a neurotransmitter that is produced from levodopa), which is then transmitted to the thalamus and cerebral cortex, modulating movement. With PD, impairment in neuronal connections and death of cells develop between the substantia nigra and the putamen of the basal ganglia, resulting in decreased levels of dopamine. Symptoms appear when 60-80% of neuronal cells are impaired and dopamine levels drop by 20-50%. As dopamine levels fall, other areas of the basal ganglia function abnormally as well, further impairing motor function. Depression is common with PD.

Alzheimer's disease

The network of neurons, branches, and synapses within the central nervous system is called the neuron forest. Electrical charges are transmitted at about 1 trillion points (synapses) with the release of neurotransmitters. In Alzheimer's disease, there is disruption in both the electrical activity and the neurotransmitters. The cerebral cortex begins to atrophy, especially in the area of the hippocampus, which controls storage of new memories, resulting in characteristic short-term memory loss. Amyloid plaques (clusters of protein fragments) form between the neurons, and as the neurons die and deteriorate, tangled strands of another protein occur. Researchers believe that these structures cause the brain damage associated with Alzheimer's disease:
- Plaques form from beta-amyloid, which is a sticky protein found in the fatty membrane surrounding neurons, and are believed to block neurotransmission or trigger an immune response.
- Tangles form when the tau protein, which supports the transport system within a neuron, begins to collapse, causing the transport system to disintegrate and the cell to die.

Stages

There are a number of methods for staging Alzheimer's disease. Staging is done by a combination of physical exam, history (often provided by family or caregivers), and mental assessment, as there is no definitive test for Alzheimer's. The 7-stage classification system (developed by Gary Reisberg, MD) is used by the Alzheimer's Association:

Stage 1	Pre-clinical with no evident impairment although slight changes may be occurring within the brain.
Stage 2	Very mild cognitive decline with some misplacing of items and forgetting things or words, but impairment is not usually noticeable to others or found on medical examination.
Stage 3	Mild, early-stage cognitive decline with short-term memory loss, problems with reading retention, remembering names, handling money, planning, and organizing. May misplace items of value.
Stage 4	Moderate cognitive decline with decreased knowledge of current affairs or family history, difficulty doing complex tasks, and social withdrawal. This stage is more easily recognized on exam and may persist for 2-10 years, during which the patients may be able to manage most activities of daily living and hygiene.

Stage 5	Moderately-severe cognitive decline as the cerebral cortex and hippocampus shrink and the ventricles enlarge. Patients are obviously confused and disoriented to date, time, and place. Patients may have difficulty using/understanding speech and managing activities of daily living. They may forget their address and telephone number. They may dress inappropriately, forget to eat resulting in weight loss, or eat a poor diet. They may be unable to do simple math, such as counting backward by 2s.
Stage 6	Moderately severe cognitive decline as the brain continues to shrink and neurons die. Patients are profoundly confused and unable to care for themselves and may undergo profound personality changes. They may confuse fiction and reality. They may fail to recognize family members, experience difficulty toileting, and begin to pace obsessively or wander away. Sundowner's syndrome, in which the person has disruption of waking/sleeping cycles and tends to get restless and wander about at night, is common. Patients may develop obsessive behaviors, such as tearing items, pulling at the hair, or wringing hands. This stage (with stage 7) may be prolonged, lasting 1-5 years.
Stage 7	Very severe cognitive decline during which most patients are wheelchair bound or bedbound and lose most ability to speak beyond a few words. They are incontinent of urine and feces and may be unable to sit unsupported or hold head up. They choke easily and have increased weakness and rigidity of muscles.

Huntington's disease

Huntington's disease is an autosomal-dominant genetic disease caused by a mutation (repeats) of the huntingtin (IT15) gene of chromosome 4. The severity of the disease relates to the number or repeats. This defect causes destruction of neurons in the basal ganglia and the cerebral cortex, especially the cerebellum. The cerebellum excites movement, and the basal ganglia inhibit it, maintaining a balance that allows smooth coordination of muscle activity. Any disruption in the system can result in unwanted movements or the inability to control movements. The putamen and caudate comprise the neostriatum (part of the basal ganglia) and these are the first neural cells to die, interfering with both direct and indirect motor pathways. Damage to the direct motor pathway causes under-stimulation of the motor cortex, resulting in slow movement. Damage to the indirect motor pathways leads to over-stimulation of the motor cortex, resulting in chorea (rapid body movements). As cells of the basal ganglia die, the cerebellum atrophies, the ventricles enlarge, and gray and white matter are reduced. Huntington's disease may cause depression, suicidal ideation, mood swings, and memory loss.

Non-Alzheimer's dementias

- Creutzfeld-Jakob disease: This causes rapidly progressive dementia with impaired memory, behavioral changes, and incoordination.
- Dementia with Lewy Bodies: Cognitive and physical decline is similar to Alzheimer's, but symptoms may fluctuate frequently. This form of dementia may include visual hallucinations, muscle rigidity, and tremors.

- Fronto-temporal dementia: This may cause marked changes in personality and behavior and is characterized by difficulty using and understanding language.
- Mixed dementia: Dementia mirrors Alzheimer's and another type because of 2 different causes of dementia.
- Normal pressure hydrocephalus: This is characterized by ataxia, memory loss, and urinary incontinence.
- Parkinson's dementia: This form of dementia may involve impaired decision making, and difficulty concentrating, learning new material, understanding complex language, and sequencing.
- Inflexibility. Short or long-term memory loss may occur.
- Vascular dementia: Memory loss may be less pronounced than that common to Alzheimer's, but symptoms are similar.

Brainstem

The brainstem (connecting the spinal cord and the cerebrum) comprises masses of gray matter and nerve fibers, is located at the base of the brain, and controls most autonomic functions, including breathing, arousal, digestion, and heart rate. The brainstem contains the following structures:
- Midbrain: Connects the spinal cord to other brain regions and contains reflex centers to move the head and eyes and maintain balance.
- Medulla oblongata: Elongation of the spinal cord extending to the pons. Conducts impulses to and from the brain and spinal cord and contains centers to control the heart and respirations.
- Pons: Bulging area that is found on the underside of the brainstem. It carries impulses between the medulla oblongata and the cerebrum and also controls the rate of breathing.

Cerebellum and basal ganglia

The cerebellum, below the occipital lobes, comprises 2 hemispheres connected by the vermis. The cerebellum is primarily white matter with a thin covering of gray matter (cerebellar cortex). Three nerve tracts in the cerebellum carry sensory information from the spinal cord to the rest of the central nervous system. The cerebellum processes information about actual body position and desired position and sends motor impulses based on the information to facilitate balance and coordinate movement. The basal ganglia (masses of gray matter in the cerebral hemispheres) mediate voluntary movement and coordination and play a role in cognition. The basal ganglia are located in the telencephalon region of the brain, and the corpus striatum, subthalamic nucleus, substantia nigra are all components of the basal ganglia. The corpus striatum (caudate nucleus and lenticular nucleus) comprises alternating layers of white and gray matter that mediate movement and executive function. The substantia nigra regulates mood, produces the neurotransmitter dopamine, and mediates voluntary movement.

Diencephalon

The diencephalon is located above the brainstem and between the cerebral hemispheres. It comprises primarily gray matter and surrounds the third ventricle. The diencephalon contains a number of structures:
- Thalamus: Receives sensory input from other parts of the central nervous system (CNS) and carries them to appropriate areas of the cerebral cortex. The thalamus serves as a gateway and also an editor for sensory input (except for smell).

- Hypothalamus: Regulates heart rate, blood pressure, temperature, fluid and electrolyte balance, hunger, weight, stomach and intestines, and sleep and also produces substances that stimulate the pituitary gland to release hormones.
- Optic chiasm: The optic nerves cross in this area anterior to the pituitary gland.
- Posterior pituitary gland: Stores and secretes oxytocin and antidiuretic hormone, which are produced by the hypothalamus.
- Mammillary bodies: Active in memory of smells.
- Pineal gland: Attached to the third ventricle, produces melatonin, and mediates sleep.

Cerebrum

The cerebrum comprises 2 cerebral hemispheres connected by the corpus callosum and is further divided into lobes. The cerebrum is primarily white matter composed of myelinated nerve fibers with a thin layer of gray matter called the cerebral cortex. The frontal lobes mediate reasoning, higher mental processes, problem solving, motor function, memory, and judgment. Broca's area in the left frontal lobe is essential to communication, both in understanding language and mediating facial nerves and expression. The occipital lobes control vision and recognition, and the parietal lobes mediate sensory function, cognition, and understanding speech. The temporal lobes regulate emotion, memory, hearing, and some functions of speech, and also interpret sensory experiences, visual pictures, and music. Wernicke's area is located in the left temporal lobe and is responsible for language comprehension.

Limbic system

The limbic system, in the region of the diencephalon, is essential to regulation of emotion, hormones, mood, and pain/pleasure sensations. The limbic system is comprised of several structures, including:
- Amygdala: An almond-shaped grouping of nuclei responsible for mediating arousal, emotion and fear responses, and hormones.
- Cingulate gyrus: The structure responsible for matching sensory input with emotional response.
- Hippocampus: A group of neurons responsible for organizing and processing memories, spatial relationships, and emotional regulation.
- Hypothalamus: A structure that is involved in almost all body processes, including autonomic functions, emotions, homeostasis, endocrine and sleep regulation, and others.
- Thalamus: A group of cells that mediates motor function, and receives, processes, and relays sensory signals.

Pituitary gland

The pituitary gland, part of the endocrine system but controlled by the brain, is located at the base of the brain inferior to the optic chiasm and is attached to the hypothalamus. The posterior lobe, primarily nerve fibers, stores and releases oxytocin and antidiuretic hormone, produced by the hypothalamus, which sends nerve impulses to the posterior pituitary to stimulate release of hormones. The anterior lobe, enclosed in a dense capsule and containing glandular tissue, secretes numerous hormones, including growth hormone (somatotropin), adrenocorticotropic hormone (ACTH), thyroid-stimulating hormone (TSH), follicle-stimulating hormone (FSH), luteinizing hormone (LH), and prolactin (which promotes milk production). Instead of nerve impulses, the hypothalamus produces releasing hormones that stimulate the pituitary to release specific hormones and other hormones that inhibit release of pituitary hormones.

Ventricular system

The brain's ventricular system protects the various structures of the brain from traumatic injury while transporting cerebrospinal fluid. There are 5 structures of the ventricular system:
1. The aqueduct of Sylvius (a cerebrospinal fluid channel between the third and fourth ventricles).
2. Choroid plexus (produces cerebrospinal fluid and acts as a buffer between the fluid and blood).
3. Third ventricle (another channel for cerebrospinal fluid).
4. Fourth ventricle (between the pons and medulla, acts as the primary channel for fluid to the spinal cord).
5. Lateral ventricle (the final channel for cerebrospinal fluid).

Serotonin

Serotonin is 1 of the 4 major neurotransmitters. Serotonin affects a variety of mood and physical disorders, including depression, psychosis, anxiety, nausea and vomiting, migraines, and other ailments. Serotonin affects many aspects of mood and physical health, and this neurotransmitter is a mediator of mood, sleep, sexual desire, anger, and appetite. The serotonin neurotransmitter system originates in the caudal dorsal raphe nucleus and the rostral dorsal raphe nucleus. Axons of the serotonin neurons originating in these areas of the raphe nucleus terminate in various areas of the brain and central nervous system, including the spinal cord, cerebral cortex, thalamus, striatum, hypothalamus, cingulate gyrus, neocortex, hippocampus, and amygdala.

Dopamine

Dopamine is 1 of the 4 major neurotransmitters. Dopamine affects a variety of mood and cognitive disorders, including bipolar disorder, attention-deficit/hyperactivity disorders, anxiety disorders, psychosis, and others. This system is primarily responsible for mediating the motor system, reward/pleasure system, and cognition. Dopamine is a stabilizing force in the brain, regulating the flow of impulses, but it does not cross the blood-brain barrier so all action is in the brain. Dopamine also affects endocrine function and may play a role in mediating nausea. There are 4 major dopamine pathways in the brain: the mesocortical pathway, mesolimbic pathway, nigrostriatal pathway, and tuberoinfundibular pathway. These pathways originate in the hypothalamus, substantia nigra, and ventral tegmentum. Parkinson's disease is characterized by inadequate production of dopamine.

Glutamate and GABA, monoamines, and neuropeptides

Glutamate and GABA (gamma-aminobutyric acid) are fast-acting neurotransmitters that are able to process received signals within just a few milliseconds. GABA has an inhibitory function, meaning it occupies and "stops" neurons. Glutamate stimulates and "turns on" neuronal action after meeting with a dendrite. Both types of neurotransmitters have the ability to quickly influence chemical signaling within the central nervous system. Thus, both glutamate and GABA are key elements in psychopharmacological treatments.
Monoamines and neuropeptides are neurotransmitters; but, unlike glutamate and GABA, these neurotransmitters are slow acting and may take as many as several seconds to process and

transmit neurotransmissions. Because of their slow onset of action, monoamines and neuropeptides are also called neuromodulators. Since a neuron can only process information as fast as the slowest signal it receives, neuromodulators control the entire pace of signal transmission. Monoamines and neuropeptides can be either excitatory or inhibitory. The type of signal they modulate and the design of the specific neurotransmitter determine function.

Acetylcholine

Acetylcholine is a 1 of the 4 major neurotransmitters. Acetylcholine plays a role in a variety of cognitive and neurodegenerative disorders, including attention-deficit/hyperactivity disorders, Alzheimer's disease, and other dementias. Acetylcholine is active in the central and peripheral nervous systems. Acetylcholine, the neurotransmitter released by a cholinergic synapse, affects learning, short-term memory, arousal, and pleasure/reward systems. Moreover, the parasympathetic nervous system (the visceral nerves of the autonomic nervous system comprising part of the peripheral nervous system) is completely cholinergic, and acetylcholine transmits impulses that activate muscles. The cholinergic neurotransmitter system originates in the basal optic nucleus of Meynert, the medial septal nucleus, and the pontomesencephalotegmental complex.

Gene, alleles, genome, genotype, and phenotype

- Genes: The basic biological unit of inheritance. A gene is a section of deoxyribonucleic acid (DNA) that contains the equation for specific cell formation and building. Genes are found in specific sites on the chromosomes.
- Alleles: One or more alternate forms of a gene.
- Genome: The complete person's genes and alleles, containing all hereditary factors.
- Genotype: The sum of a person's genetic constitution and alleles. One's genotype is unique to the individual and determines the type species.
- Phenotype: The observable characteristics or behaviors (physical, biochemical, and physiological) of an individual. Physical characteristics include height, weight, and eye color. Likewise, the phenotype may include one's expressions, responses to stimuli, and other behaviors. Phenotype is influenced by both genetics and environment.

Neuron

Neurons are nerve cells that transmit nerve impulses throughout the central and peripheral nervous systems for the brain to interpret. The neuron includes the cell body or soma, the dendrites, and the axons. The soma contains the nucleus. The nucleus contains the chromosomes. The dendrite extends from the cell body and resembles the branches of a tree. The dendrite receives chemical messages from other cells across the synapse, a small gap. The axon is a thread-like extension of the cell body, up to 3 feet long in spinal nerves. The axon transmits an electro-chemical message along its length to another cell. Axons of neurons in the peripheral nervous system (PNS) that deal with muscles are myelinated with fat to speed up the transmission of messages. Neurons in the PNS that deal with pain are unmyelinated because transmission does not have to be fast. Some neurons in the central nervous system (CNS) are myelinated by oligodendrocytes.

Spinal cord

The spinal cord carries the nerves from the brain to the peripheral nervous system, contains the cerebrospinal fluid, and is covered with 3 protective membranes (meninges) that are continuous around the brain and spinal cord. The spinal cord contains a number of structures:

- Pia mater, the innermost layer, adheres to the spinal cord.
- Subarachnoid space, between the pia mater and arachnoid mater (the next layer), contains the cerebrospinal fluid. Spinal (subarachnoid) anesthesia is administered into this space.
- Arachnoid mater is the primary impermeable barrier preventing movement of drugs from the epidural to the subarachnoid space. It is closely adherent to the dura mater (outside layer).
- Dura mater is a protective fibroelastic membrane that is fairly impenetrable.
- Epidural space lies outside of the dura mater and contains lymphatics, fatty tissue, nerve roots, small arteries, and the epidural venous plexus. Epidural and caudal anesthesia is administered into this space. The (adult) depth ranges from 6 mm at L2 and 4-5 mm in the mid-thoracic area.

Central nervous system

The components of the central nervous system (CNS) are the brain and spinal cord. The CNS is the largest portion of the nervous system. The CNS is housed in the dorsal cavity, which includes the cranial cavity (the skull) and the spinal cavity (the vertebral column and spinal cord). The brain is responsible for behavior, and the spinal cord mediates signals traveling to and from the brain. The major sections of the brain include the brainstem, the cerebral hemispheres (comprising the frontal lobes, temporal lobes, occipital lobes, and parietal lobes), and the cerebellum. The major sections of the spinal cord include cervical nerves and vertebrae, thoracic nerves and vertebrae, lumbar nerves and vertebrae, and the sacral nerves and vertebrae. In addition to the nerves and vertebrae, the spinal column is also made up of vertebral discs, which serve to cushion the vertebrae.

Somatic nervous system

The somatic nervous system comprises cranial and spinal nerves that connect the central nervous system to the skeletal muscles and skin. The somatic nervous system is the voluntarily-controlled component of the peripheral nervous system, and it receives and responds to external sensory stimuli from the skin and sensory organs. Efferent nerves mediate movement through stimulation of skeletal muscles, allowing the person to move. The somatic nervous system carries sensations of pain to the brain, helping the individual avoid danger, so it's part of the protective system of the body. Somatic nerves leave the spinal column as nerve roots and may form a plexus or an individual nerve. Plexi include cervical, brachial, lumbosacral, and sacral. Individual nerves include the occipital, intercostal, and suprascapular.

PNS

The peripheral nervous system (PNS) comprises the long nerves that serve organs and limbs. The PNS is further divided into the autonomic nervous system and the somatic nervous system. Sympathetic nerves are part of the autonomic nervous system. Sympathetic nerves are found both within the central nervous system (CNS) (preganglionic) and the PNS (postganglionic), with those in the CNS communicating with those in the PNS through a series of ganglia by means of neurotransmitters (acetylcholine) at synapses. The sympathetic nervous system (T1-L2 or L3) activates in times of stress and is implicated in pain. The nerves innervate deep structures, viscera, and skin. Ganglia are paired: 3 cervical, 12 thoracic, 4 lumbar, 4 sacral, and 1 impar (at coccyx). The parasympathetic nerves maintain a state of homeostasis when the body is not under stress. The autonomic nervous system mediates the body's organs and maintains homeostasis. Functions of the autonomic nervous system include heart rate and function, respiration, digestion, sexual arousal, and other systems.

Noradrenaline and norepinephrine

Noradrenaline is also called norepinephrine. It is 1 of the 4 major neurotransmitters in the brain, released by the adrenal glands. Noradrenaline is primarily responsible for mediating arousal and the reward system, and is released in response to stress. This noradrenaline system originates in the locus coeruleus and lateral tegmental field, and it is able to transmit messages to both sides of the brain. Axons from neurons firing in the locus coeruleus and lateral tegmental field act on adrenergic receptors in the spinal cord, thalamus, hypothalamus, hippocampus, amygdala, neocortex, striatum, cingulate gyrus, and other areas. Norepinephrine plays a role in depressive disorders and attention-deficit/hyperactivity disorders, among others.

Areas of the brain associated with aggression, anger, and violence

The 3 main areas of the brain associated with altered aggression, anger, and violence include the limbic system, frontal lobes, and the hypothalamus:
- The *limbic system* is involved with the processing of information, memory, and emotions. The area known as the amygdale is particularly involved in the expression of rage and fear. Alterations in this system may result in altered levels of anger and violence.
- The *frontal lobes* are involved with reasoning and intentional behaviors. Trauma to this area of the brain can lead to personality changes, angry emotional outbursts, or impaired decision-making abilities.
- The *hypothalamus* is involved with the body's stress-response system. This area of the brain sends messages to the pituitary gland to raise steroid levels within the body in response to stress. Malfunctions of the hypothalamus can lead to over-stimulation and abnormally elevated levels of steroids.

Diathesis-stress model

The diathesis-stress model is a theoretical psychological principal in which genes and environment interact to bring about mental illness. In other words, mental illness is a product of both nature and nurture. The diathesis-stress model theorizes that in the presence of genetic predisposition, environmental stress may trigger mental illness. The intensity of the stress and the severity of genetic predisposition may vary. For example, someone who has a weak genetic predisposition for mental illness may only develop the illness if he/she is exposed to extreme stress. On the other hand, an individual who has a strong genetic predisposition for mental illness may develop illness in the presence of a little stress. It is important to note, however, that an individual may have underlying genetic predisposition for mental illness but may never develop illness, regardless of stress.

Alcohol withdrawal

Chronic abuse of ethanol (alcoholism) is associated with alcohol withdrawal syndrome (delirium tremens) with abrupt cessation of alcohol intake, resulting in hallucinations, tachycardia, diaphoresis, and sometimes-psychotic behavior. It may be precipitated by trauma or infection and has a high mortality rate, 5-15% with treatment and 35% without treatment. Management includes:

- Monitor vital signs and blood gases.
- Use the Clinical Instrument for Withdrawal for Alcohol (CIWA) to measure symptoms of withdrawal.
- Assess and monitor level of consciousness, orientation, alterations in sensory impressions, agitation, and anxiety.
- Provide an environment with minimal sensory stimulus (lower lights, close blinds).
- Implement fall and seizure precautions.
- Provide nutritional support and monitor intake and output.
- Implement measures to assure proper sleep and stress management.
- Express acceptance and reassurance.
- Maintain body temperature.

People easily aroused can usually safely sleep off the effects of ingesting too much alcohol but if semi-conscious or unconscious, emergency medical treatment (such as intravenous fluids and medications, intubation, and/or dialysis) may be necessary.

Physiologic response to stress and anxiety

The physiologic response to stress and anxiety occurs on a continuum from mild to severe. These responses are not controllable by the person experiencing these feelings and are mediated through the immune and autonomic nervous systems. The sympathetic nervous system turns on the physiologic response to stress and anxiety and readies the body to react. Under stress, the hypothalamus acts to stimulate the pituitary gland to secrete a hormone, which leads to increased cortisol levels. This increased production may lead to elevated availability of glucose for heightened cellular metabolism. In some individuals the parasympathetic nervous system can dominate during stress. The associated symptoms often have the opposite effect of what is seen when the sympathetic nervous system is in control. Cardiovascular responses can include decreased blood pressure and heart rate, feelings of faintness, or actual fainting. There can also be an increased need to urinate along with feelings of abdominal pain, nausea, and diarrhea.

Effects of stress and the sympathetic nervous

The sympathetic nervous system releases epinephrine in response to stress and anxiety. This affects the cardiovascular and respiratory systems by revving up their normal responses and readying the body to fly into action. In the cardiovascular system, the heart rate and blood pressure increase with associated feelings of palpitations. Blood is shunted away from non-vital organs, such as the stomach, intestines, and kidneys, resulting in decreased peristalsis and urine output. There is increased blood flow to necessary muscle groups to encourage a quick response time. Blood coagulation time increases. In the respiratory system, there is an increase in the rate of respirations and a decrease in the depth of respirations; breathing becomes rapid and shallow and is associated with feelings of shortness of air.

In response to stress, the sympathetic nervous system usually leads to a decrease in blood flow in the gastrointestinal (GI) tract. This decreases appetite and movement of the intestinal tract. The neuromuscular system is charged up and ready to respond. Reflex time is increased, and there can be some twitching or shaking of muscles. The need for sleep is greatly reduced, leading to periods of insomnia. The facial expression may be tense and anxious, and the patient may actually pace about. The patient may have uncontrolled muscle movements, restlessness, fast speech, avoidance, or startle easily. The integumentary system also responds. The skin may become flushed or itchy and there is an increase in sweat gland production. These reactions can lead to ineffective interpersonal communication or social withdrawal. Cognitive functioning can also be affected by stress and anxiety. The patient might appear distracted or unable to concentrate, forgetful, confused, or make errors in judgment not normally seen. The patient may also experience flashbacks or have frightening hallucinations.

Hallucinations

Different types of hallucinations include:
- Auditory: This is the most common type of hallucination and often involves patients' hearing voices or commands to action, but some patients may hear music, clicks, or other sounds, which may be very persistent.
- Visual: Patients may believe that they see people or other things, such as bugs or snakes, which are not present. In some cases visual hallucinations may be of unformed images, such as bright or flashing lights, or distortions.
- Gustatory: Patients may experience bad tastes.
- Olfactory: Patients may complain of smells that are not present, especially noxious or unpleasant smells.
- Tactile: Patients may feel as though something is touching them or crawling on their skin.
- Hallucinogen-induced: Various hallucinations may occur within a short time (minutes to an hour) of ingesting a hallucinogen, such as LSD.
- Schizophrenia-induced: During psychotic episodes, patient may experience a variety of hallucinations.

Neurological examination of brain function

Brain function can be inferred from the neurological exam:
- General appearance: Includes posture, affect, dysmorphic features, involuntary motor movements, and tremors. Resting tumors suggest impairment of the substantia nigra; and volitional tremors, cerebellar damage.
- Mental status exam: Evaluates cognitive processes, including speech and thought, and cerebellum function. Personality changes may indicate damage to frontal lobes.
- Cranial nerve exam (I-XII): Evaluates sensorium (hearing, taste, smell, vision) and swallowing as well as muscles of the face and speech. Abnormalities point to possible lesions in the area of the specific nerve.
- Motor system (position, involuntary motor activity, muscle strength/tone): Helps to identify lesions of the upper motor neurons and lower motor neurons depending on the type of abnormalities with upper characterized by hyperreflexia and spasticity and lower by hypotonia and hyporeflexia.
- Sensory (sense of position, touch, pain): Helps to identify neuropathy and impaired sensations. Abnormalities may help pinpoint damage to the sensory cortex located in the parietal lobe.

- Reflexes: Show abnormalities of C5-C7, L3-L4, and S1.
- Coordination and gait: Abnormalities may be indicative of neurological disease (multiple sclerosis, Parkinson's disease) or cerebellar lesions.

Hypernatremia

Hypernatremia is excess salt, indicated by a serum sodium level greater than 145 mEq/L. In bedridden seniors, hyponatremia can be from lack of access to water. Other causes of hypernatremia are: Too much sodium in IV fluid; too much salt in the diet; too much Mannitol; glycosuria; inadequate water intake due to a defective thirst mechanism from a hypothalamic problem; excessive water loss from sweating, vomiting and diarrhea; burns; and diabetes insipidus. Patients present with thirst, signs of dehydration, lethargy and weakness, and seizures or coma in severe cases. Base your diagnosis on the history, physical exam and serum sodium level. Normal sodium ranges between136 to 145 mEq/L. Replace the free water deficit. The free water deficit = total body water (TBW) × [(plasma Na/140) – 1]. The total body water is the patient's weight in kilograms multiplied by 0.6. Free water replacement can be accomplished orally in conscious patients who can swallow or intravenously in more seriously ill patients.

Hyponatremia

Hyponatremia is lack of salt, indicated by a plasma sodium less than 135 mEq/L. Hyponatremia can be from severe dehydration, but is usually secondary to some other disorder. Hyponatremia can be hypervolemic, euvolemic or hypovolemic. This is determined by calculating the plasma osmolality and volume status of the patient. The Biochemistry lab calculates the plasma osmolality as follows: Plasma osmolality = (2 × Na$^+$) + (BUN/2.8) + (glucose/18). Causes of hyponatremia include kidney disease, excess free water intake, diuretics, SIADH, severe vomiting or diarrhea, low-sodium diet, liver disease and congestive heart failure. Symptoms depend on the acuity and severity of hyponatremia. Patients may be asymptomatic. Symptoms can include nausea, vomiting, headache and confusion. Severe cases can present with seizures and coma. Order serum electrolytes, BUN, glucose, and urine sodium (UNa). Be concerned if plasma sodium is <135 mEq/L; death often occurs below 105 mEq/L. Treatment depends on volume status and underlying cause of the hyponatremia.

Needs of Alzheimer's or dementia patients

The needs of the patient with Alzheimer's disease or dementia will vary depending on the stage of the disorder, but by the time the patient has moderate disease, some needs are evident:
- Safety: Because patients may wander and may have impaired judgment, safety issues are a primary concern. Patients may need movement or door alarms and locks on outside doors. Knives, scissors and other dangerous tools may need to be removed.
- Nutritional support: Patients often forget they've eaten and eat again or forget to eat, so supervision of nutrition is necessary. Patients are often unable to shop or prepare food.
- Assistance with ADLs and IADLs: Patients may need assistance with all ADLs, especially those related to personal hygiene. They may also need assistance with all IADLs and may need a conservator if no family is available to assist.
- Exercise: Patients need to remain active. Walking is an ideal exercise as patients often pace.
- Emotional support: Patients need and often respond to love and kindness.

Needs of traumatic brain injury patients

The needs of the patient with a traumatic brain injury depend on the extent of the damage but problems and interventions can include:
- Impaired verbal communication: Speech therapy and communication enhancement approaches.
- Impaired physical mobility: Physical therapy, assistive devices, and occupational therapy.
- Impaired bowel/urinary elimination: Bowel/bladder training, and assistance with toileting.
- Disturbed thought processes: Memory training, medications, safety precautions, cognitive stimulation, and behavioral therapy.
- Disturbed sensory perceptions: Nutritional and environmental management and hearing and vision support.
- Insomnia: Environmental management and sleep enhancement techniques.
- Impaired swallowing: Swallowing therapy.
- Risk for injury: Safety precautions, seizure precautions, and seizure prophylaxis.
- Impaired parenting skills: Parenting classes and child protection strategies.
- Delayed growth and development: Monitoring and enhancement strategies.
- Substance abuse: Intervention, 12-step programs and support programs.
- Risk for violence: Intervention, behavioral therapy, and family therapy.
- Risk for suicide: Monitoring, support groups, therapy, and medications.

Pharmacokinetics

Pharmacokinetics relates to the effects that the body has on a drug, and pharmacodynamics relates to the effects that a drug has on the body. Both must be considered to ensure adequate dosing to achieve the optimal response from medications. With all drugs there is an intake (dose) and a response. Pharmacokinetics relates to the route of administration, the absorption, the dosage, the frequency of administration, the distribution, and the serum levels achieved over time. The drug's rate of clearance (elimination) and doses needed to ensure therapeutic benefit must be considered. Most drugs are cleared through the kidneys, with water-soluble compounds excreted more readily than protein-soluble compounds. Volume of distribution (intravenous [IV] drug dose divided by plasma concentration) determines the rate at which the drug passes into tissue. Drug distribution depends on the degree of protein binding and ion trapping that takes place.

Half-time, recovery time, and effect-site equilibrium
Elimination half-time is the time needed to reduce plasma concentrations to 50% during elimination. Usually the equivalent of 5 half-times is needed to completely eliminate a drug. Five half-times are also needed to achieve steady-state plasma concentrations if giving doses intermittently. Context-sensitive half-time, in contrast, is the time needed to reach a specific amount of decrease (50%, 60%) after stopping administration of a drug. Recovery time is the length of time it takes for plasma levels to decrease to the point that the person awakens. This is affected by plasm concentration. Effect-site equilibrium is the time between administration of a drug and clinical effect (the point at which the drug reaches the appropriate receptors) and must be considered when determining dose, time, and frequency of anesthetic agents. The bioavailability of drugs may vary, depending upon the degree of metabolism that takes place before the drug reaches its site of action.

Pharmacodynamics

Pharmacodynamics relates to biological effects (therapeutic or adverse) of drug administration over time. Drug transport, absorption, means of elimination, and half-life must all be considered when determining effects. Responses may include continuous responses, such as blood pressure variations, or dichotomous response, in which an event either occurs or does not (such as death). Information from pharmacodynamics provides feedback to modify medication dosage (pharmacokinetics). Drugs provide biological effects primarily by interacting with receptor sites (specific protein molecules) in the cell membrane. Receptors include voltage-sensitive ion channels (sodium, chloride, potassium, and calcium channels), ligand-gated ion channels, and transmembrane receptors. Agonist drugs exert effects after binding with a receptor while antagonist drugs bind with a receptor but have no effects, so they can block agonists from binding. The total number of receptors may vary, up-regulating or down-regulating in response to stimuli (such as drug administration). Dose-response curves show the relationship between the amount of drug given and the resultant plasma concentration and biological effects.

Tolerance, dependency, and withdrawal

A patient can develop a tolerance to a particular medication when that medication is used over a period of time. The effects of the medication diminish and can lead to a need to increase the dosage to achieve the same response. Some diagnoses, such as schizophrenia, require medications throughout the patient's life, so changing medications may become necessary. Sometimes dependency and withdrawal symptoms can be seen along with the development of tolerance. Dependency can be psychological or physical in nature. The withdrawal of this medication can produce stress or anxiety along with real physical symptoms. The medication will often have to be weaned by slowly decreasing the dosage. In severe cases, abrupt discontinuation of the medication can lead to death.

Pharmaceutical treatment

Trial period of new medication
When initiating any sort of pharmaceutical treatment, it is important to have an adequate trial period for each therapy before switching to alternative therapies due to unresponsiveness. Generally speaking, a medication is tested for 8 weeks before switching. However, 4 to 6 weeks is sufficient for stimulants before opting for a second-line treatment. Before switching medications, one should check with a pharmacist to ensure the dose of the current therapy has been optimized. It is not uncommon for agents to be prescribed in doses that fail to optimize the drug. Drug optimization may occur at either a lower or higher dose for an individual patient than the dose that is commonly prescribed. Dose optimization is 1 of the many reasons why upward and downward titrations are important.

Initiation and stabilization
The phases of pharmacological treatment begin with:
- Initiation: Involves a complete assessment and patient history. Lab work includes blood chemistry, complete blood count, liver, kidney, and thyroid function tests. The choice of medication and dosage may be adjusted based on these results. The inpatient should be closely monitored with the first dose of any medication for adverse reactions.
- Stabilization: Determination of the proper dosage of medication, with increases or decreases to achieve the desired response with minimal side effects. There should be an ongoing assessment process, including physical and psychological assessments along with

re-evaluation of certain lab values or drug levels. The patient should be closely monitored for any unwanted side effects, drug interactions, or adverse reactions such as abnormal muscle movements or elevated blood pressure or temperature. The initial medication chosen may not produce the desired response, and a second drug may be added or a drug may be discontinued altogether.

<u>Maintenance and discontinuation</u>
The last 2 phases of pharmacological treatment include:
- Maintenance: Utilizing medication to prevent reoccurrence of unwanted symptoms. Symptoms may reappear because of a change in metabolism caused by the medication, development of tolerance, physical illness, stress, or use of additional prescription or over the counter medications. Some side effects may not be evident until the patient has been on the medication for a period of time. Patients must be educated about potential side effects and possible decrease in the drug's efficacy and able to recognize red-flag signs and symptoms. Patients should understand the importance of follow-up visits and testing to evaluate their particular medication regimen.
- Discontinuation: Stopping medication. Most psychiatric medications are not stopped abruptly, but the dosage is slowly decreased over time. During the weaning period, the patient should be closely monitored for reappearance of the unwanted symptoms. Weaning helps to avoid withdrawal symptoms. Support, reassurance, and education are vital to the successful discontinuation of many psychiatric medications.

Gerontological pharmacology

There are a number of issues that can affect gerontological pharmacology:
- Antidepressants are associated with excess sedation, so typical doses are only 16-33% of a younger adult's dose. Selective serotonin reuptake inhibitors (SSRIs) are safest, but Prozac® may cause anorexia, anxiety, and insomnia so should be avoided.
- Older antipsychotics, such as haloperidol, have high incidence of side effects. Atypical antipsychotics appear to be safer with risperidone (<2 mg daily) having the fewest adverse effects. The lowest possible doses should be tried first with careful monitoring of any antipsychotic.
- Adverse effects of drugs are 2-3 times more common in older adults than younger adults, often related to polypharmacy.
- Drug and nutrient interactions may impact nutrition by impairing appetite. Interactions may also alter the pharmacokinetics of nutrients or drugs, interfering with absorption, distribution, metabolism, and elimination.

Pediatric pharmacology

There are a number of pediatric pharmacology concerns. Pediatric doses are calculated according to the child's weight in kilograms, but other factors may affect dosage. Weight is estimated by age (although actual weight is safer):

50th percentile weight (kg) = (Age X 2) + 9.

Only pediatric medications should be prescribed if possible. Adult pills, for example, should not be cut for use for a child as even small variations in dosage may have adverse effects. Dosage should always be checked. Drug therapy in children may sometimes require adult dosages due to children's increased ability to quickly metabolize the medications. Children may also exhibit unusual responses or side effects to drugs compared to adults and should be very closely evaluated and frequently assessed.

Anaphylaxis syndrome

Anaphylaxis syndrome is a sudden acute systemic immunoglobulin E (IgE) or non-immunoglobulin E (non-IgE) inflammatory response affecting the cardiopulmonary and other systems.
- IgE-mediated response (anaphylactic shock) is an antibody-antigen reaction against an allergen, such as milk, peanuts, latex, insect bites, drugs, or fish. This is the most common type.
- Non-IgE-mediated response (anaphylactoid reaction) is a systemic reaction to infection, exercise, radio contrast material, or other triggers. While the response is almost identical to the other type, it does not involve IgE.

Typically, with IgE-mediated response, an antigen triggers release of substances, such as histamine and prostaglandins, which affect the skin, cardiopulmonary, and gastrointestinal systems. Histamine causes initial erythema and edema by inducing vasodilation. Each time the person has contact with the antigen, more antibodies form in response, and allergic reactions worsen. Anaphylactic shock related to anesthesia is rare, although anaphylactoid reactions may occur with opioids, hypnotics, and muscle relaxants. Antibiotics (penicillin, sulfonamides, cephalosporins) and latex allergy cause most medication/treatment related anaphylaxis.

Drug interactions

Drug interactions occur when 1 drug interferes with the activity of another in either the pharmacodynamics or pharmacokinetics:
- With pharmacodynamic interaction, both drugs may interact at receptor sites causing a change that result in an adverse effect or that interferes with a positive effect.
- With pharmacokinetic interaction, the ability of the drug to be absorbed and cleared is altered, so there may be delayed effects, changes in effects, or toxicity. Interactions may include problems in a number of areas. Absorption may be increased or (more commonly) decreased, usually related to the effects within the gastrointestinal system. Distribution of drugs may be affected, often because of changes in protein binding. Metabolism may be altered, often causing changes in drug concentration. Biotransformation of the drug must take place, usually in the liver and gastrointestinal system, but drug interactions can impair this process. Clearance interactions may interfere with the body's ability to eliminate a drug, usually resulting in increased concentration of the drug.

Stimulants

Stimulants are primarily used to treat attention-deficit/hyperactivity disorder (ADHD) in children and narcolepsy in adults. Commonly used stimulants include methylphenidate (Ritalin®, Concerta®), dextro methylphenidate (Focalyn®), dextroamphetamine (Dexedrine®), dextroamphetamine and amphetamine combinations (Adderall®). Magnesium pemoline (Cylert®) is used as a second- or third-line treatment because of liver toxicity. If 3 different stimulants fail to work, Wellbutrin® (bupropion), desipramine, or imipramine may be effective. Stimulants act on the central nervous system to heighten attentiveness and impulse control. Stimulant use should be accompanied by behavioral therapy for the child and training for the parents for 8 to 12 weeks. Stimulants are generally well-tolerated, though as many as 10% of patients may experience side effects, including abdominal pain, diminished appetite, nausea, vomiting, anorexia, headache, dizziness, insomnia, nervousness, changes in mood, social withdrawal, psychotic hallucinations, manic symptoms, depression, irritability, fatigue, nervous habits, and tics. Though stimulants have few drug-drug interactions, 2 are life-threatening: monoamine oxidase (MAO) inhibitors and furazolidone. Additionally, stimulants may interact with clonidine. Lowering dosage may relieve side effects.

Alzheimer's disease drugs

Treatment for Alzheimer's disease is aimed at slowing the progression of the disease and ensuring patient safety. Two types of drugs are approved by the Food and Drug Administration (FDA), but many clinical trials are taking place. In some cases 2 drugs (such as Aricept® and Namenda®) may be given. Patients must take medication daily and be monitored carefully, as some drugs may worsen symptoms in some patients so different drugs may need to be tried.

Type of Drug	Drug Type & indication	Adverse effects
Cholinesterase inhibitors (Prevents breakdown of acetylcholine, needed for learning and memory)	Donepezil (Aricept®): All stages of Alzheimer's. Rivastigmine (Exelon®): Mild to moderate disease. Galantamine (Razadyne®): Mild to moderate disease.	Nausea, vomiting, loss of appetite, and frequent bowel movements.
	Tacrine (Cognex®): Mild to moderate disease. (Rarely used)	Nausea, vomiting, and possible dam-age to the liver.
Memantine (Targets glutamate, involved in learning and memory)	Namenda®: Moderate to severe disease.	Headache, confusion, dizziness, and constipation.

St. John's wort

The use of complementary and alternative medicine for the treatment of depression is very common. One of the most widely utilized and studied herbal therapies for the treatment of depression is St. John's wort or hypericum. This particular herb is widely utilized to treat depression symptoms in both the United States and in European countries. It has shown some effectiveness in treating mild to moderate depression, anxiety disorder, insomnia or seasonal affective disorder. Medical providers should be aware if the patient is taking this herb due it's contraindications with many commonly prescribed medications, such as, birth control pills, statins used to treat hyperlipidemia, protease inhibitors, antineoplastics, selective serotonin reuptake inhibitors (SSRIs), anticonvulsants, theophylline, and anticoagulants (such as warfarin).

Herbal remedies and dietary supplements

There are literally thousands of herbal remedies and dietary supplements and myriad claims of success in treating or preventing disease, despite there being very little scientific evidence to support most claims. Many doctors recommend 1 daily multivitamin to ensure adequate vitamin intake and fish oil concentrate to reduce cholesterol, but patients often take high doses of herbal remedies and dietary supplements. This poses a number of problems. High doses of some vitamins can cause toxicity:

- Vitamin A: Headaches, loss of hair, liver damage, bone disorders, and birth defects.
- Vitamin C: Diarrhea and gastrointestinal upset.
- Vitamin D: Kidney stones, muscle weakness, and bleeding.
- Vitamin E: Inhibits action of vitamin K.
- Niacin: Liver damage, gastric ulcers, and increased serum glucose.
- Vitamin B_6: Neurological damage.

Herbal remedies often contain small amounts of agents found in drugs, so they can cause drug reactions and interactions. Also, patients often fail to inform their physicians when they are using alternative treatments.

SSRIs

Selective serotonin reuptake inhibitors (SSRIs) are antidepressant medications that block reuptake of serotonin (neurotransmitter) in the brain, increasing the extracellular level of the neurotransmitter and improving transmission. Neurotransmitters allow neurons to communicate with "messages" passed from a presynaptic cell (sender) in 1 neuron to a post-synaptic receptor (receiver) in the other. The exact means by which SSRIs relieve depression is not clear. All SSRIs have similar action but may have different chemical properties that cause various side effects, so some people tolerate 1 better than others. Side effects include nausea, weight gain, sexual dysfunction, excitation, agitation, insomnia, drowsiness, increased perspiration, headache, and diarrhea. In rare cases, serotonin syndrome may occur from high levels of serotonin from overdose or combination with monoamine oxidase (MAO) inhibitors, so SSRIs must not be taken within 2 weeks of each other. Symptoms include severe anxiety and agitation, hallucinations, confusion, blood pressure swings, fever, tachycardia, seizures, and coma. SSRIs are not addictive but abrupt cessation may trigger discontinuation syndrome (flu-like symptoms).

Lexapro® and Prozac®

Escitalopram (Lexapro®) and fluoxetine (Prozac®) are selective serotonin reuptake inhibitors (SSRIs) used for the treatment of major depression and generalized anxiety disorder (GAD), which includes severe anxiety and apprehension for ≥6 months. They demonstrated effectiveness for depression with 8 weeks of acute treatment and maintenance for 36 weeks, but efficacy beyond 8 weeks for GAD has not been studied. Lexapro® and Prozac® administered in the third trimester has been associated with neonatal complications. Side effects, cautions, and interactions are similar to Celexa® and other SSRIs, but incidence of side effects is somewhat different. The most common side effects are nausea (15-18%), somnolence (6-13%), insomnia (9-12%), but ejaculation disorders are more common (9-14%) with impotence and anorgasmia (females) (2-6%) also reported. Side effects vary depending on whether treatment is given for depression or GAD. Lexapro® is not associated with weight gain, but Prozac® is. Lexapro® may increase suicidal thoughts and behavior in children through young adults (≤24) while Prozac® affects both children and all adults.

Celexa®

Citalopram (Celexa®) is chemically unrelated to other SSRIs and is specifically used to treat acute depression for 6-8 weeks with antidepressive results up to 24 weeks. Celexa® administered in the third trimester has been associated with neonatal complications, so the medication should be tapered during the third trimester if possible. Common side effects include dry mouth (20%), increased perspiration, tremor, nausea, somnolence, insomnia, ejaculation disorder (occurring in 6%), and decreased libido and impotence (primarily affecting males). Celexa® is associated with slight weight loss rather than weight gain. Celexa® should not be taken with triptans, linezolid, St. John's Wort, lithium, other SSRIs or central nervous system drugs. Concurrent use of nonsteroidal anti-inflammatory drugs (NSAIDs) and aspirin may increase risk of gastrointestinal bleeding. Celexa® increases the risk of suicidal thinking and behavior from childhood to young adulthood (age 24). Celexa® should not be used to treat depressive episodes of bipolar disease.

Zoloft®

Sertraline (Zoloft®) is a selective serotonin reuptake inhibitor (SSRI) that is used for treatment of major depression, obsessive-compulsive disorder, panic disorder, post-traumatic stress disorder, premenstrual dysphoric disorder, and social anxiety disorder. Cautions and interactions are similar to other SSRIs, and side effects are similar to Paxil®. The most common side effects include headache (25%), nausea, diarrhea (20%), somnolence, insomnia, dry mouth, decreased libido (6%), and ejaculatory failure (14%). Zoloft® may increase suicidal thoughts and actions in both children and adults, especially in children <18. Zoloft® is not approved for bipolar disorder and may exacerbate the manic stage. Zoloft® is approved for pediatric patients only for treatment of obsessive-compulsive disorder (OCD), although it has been used successfully in clinical trials. Zoloft® is associated with weight loss, which may rarely be pronounced in patients, but usually averages 1-2 pounds.

Paxil®

Paroxetine (Paxil®) is a selective serotonin reuptake inhibitor (SSRI) that is used as a psychotropic drug for the treatment of major depression, obsessive-compulsive disorder (OCD), panic disorder, social anxiety disorder, generalized anxiety disorder (GAD), and post-traumatic stress disorder (PTSD); it has broader uses than some other SSRIs. Paxil® has been shown to be effective for treatment up to 1 year and is used longer for chronic conditions, such as OCD. Cautions and interactions are similar to other SSRIs, but side effects are more pronounced than with other drugs and vary depending upon the diagnosis for which treatment is given. Paxil® is approved for adult use but not for pediatrics. Paxil® may increase suicidal thoughts and actions. Weight gain is common as is headache, asthenia, nausea, dry mouth, constipation, sweating, somnolence, insomnia, and diarrhea. Ejaculatory disorders (13-28%) and decreased libido (males) (6-15%) are fairly common, with sexual dysfunction affecting females to a lesser degree.

Tricyclic antidepressants

Tricyclic antidepressants (named for the 3-ring chemical structure of the first of this group) inhibit the uptake of neurotransmitters, primarily norepinephrine and serotonin, and serve as antagonists to dopamine and histamine. Tricyclic antidepressants usually target 2 or 3 of these neurotransmitters while newer antidepressants, such as selective serotonin reuptake inhibitors (SSRIs), target only one. Tricyclic antidepressants treat depression, attention-deficit/hyperactivity disorder (ADHD), nocturnal enuresis, and pain (migraine). They are sometimes referred to as cyclic antidepressants because newer drugs have a 4-ring structure. Tricyclic antidepressants are lipophilic and highly protein-bound, so they absorb rapidly. They affect the limbic system,

Copyright © Mometrix Media. You have been licensed one copy of this document for personal use only. Any other reproduction or redistribution is strictly prohibited. All rights reserved.

decreasing β-receptors, which are stimulated by increased levels of norepinephrine, which interferes with receptor function. They have long half-lives, which increases toxic effects with overdose, and anticholinergic (primarily muscarinic) effects. Because of this, cyclic antidepressants tend to have more side effects than newer antidepressants: dry mouth, blurring vision, cardiac abnormalities, constipation, urinary retention, and hyperthermia. Alterations in memory and cognition, drowsiness, anxiety, muscle twitches, gynecomastia, and breast enlargement may occur. They are contraindicated with monoamine oxidase (MAO) inhibitors and cimetidine.

Elavil and Tofranil

Amitriptyline (Elavil®) is a tricyclic (cyclic) antidepressant that targets norepinephrine, serotonin, and histamine. It should not be taken with monoamine oxidase (MAO) inhibitors, epinephrine, or alcohol. Alcohol inhibits antidepressive action but potentiates sedation. It is used for depression, insomnia, chronic pain, and fibromyalgia. It may increase suicidal thinking, and should be used with caution for those with history of seizures, cardiac disease, thyroid disease, prostate enlargement, pregnancy, and glaucoma. It is not recommended for children under 12 years old and is not approved for bipolar disorder. It may trigger psychosis in schizophrenic patients. Imipramine (Tofranil®) targets the same neurotransmitters as amitriptyline (norepinephrine, serotonin, and histamine) and is used to treat endogenous depression (as opposed to depression caused by external factors, such as loss of job or loved one) and enuresis in children. Cautions, contraindications, and side effects are similar to amitriptyline, but extreme caution should be used with those with cardiovascular disease because of serious complications.

Norpramin, Aventyl, and Pamelor

Desipramine (Norpramin®), a metabolite of imipramine, is a tricyclic (cyclic) antidepressant that targets norepinephrine and blocks pain signals, so it is used for depression, attention-deficit/hyperactivity disorder (ADHD), and neuropathic pain. It may be used in adolescents but should not be used for younger children. Cautions, contraindications, and side effects are similar to other tricyclic antidepressants. It is contraindicated with monoamine oxidase (MAO) inhibitors and in the recovery period of a myocardial infarction (MI). It should be discontinued prior to elective surgery because of possible cardiac effects and hypertension. Nortriptyline (Aventyl®, Pamelor®), similar to desipramine, targets only norepinephrine. It is indicated only for the use of endogenous depression and is not recommended for children. Cautions, contraindications, and side effects are similar to other tricyclic antidepressants. It may exacerbate psychosis in those with schizophrenia. It may be given with electroshock therapy but should be discontinued before elective surgery.

Clinical MAO inhibitors

Monoamine oxidase (MAO) inhibitors are older antidepressant medications that are used less frequently now that others are available because they have significant side effects and interactions with other medications. MAO is an enzyme that breaks down neurotransmitters (norepinephrine, dopamine, serotonin, tyramine, and phenylethylamine) in the central nervous system. When levels of neurotransmitters fall, this can result in depression, so MAO inhibitors block this action. Selective MAO inhibitors may target only some neurotransmitters while non-selective may target all, including other enzymes. Non-selective MAO inhibitors include phenelzine (Nardil®), isocarboxazid (Marplan®), and tranylcypromine (Parnate®). People using MAO inhibitors must avoid foods with high levels of tyramine (cheeses, wines, pickles) as well as medications, such as decongestants, in order to prevent severe hypertension crises. Other side effects include tremors, orthostatic hypotension, urinary retention, muscle spasms, jaundice, and agitation. Reactions may occur with opioids as well, especially meperidine (Demerol®), resulting in hyperthermia, seizures, and coma. Patients do not need to stop medication prior to surgery.

Lithium

Lithium carbonate (Eskalith®, Lithobid®) is used to control the manic episodes associated with bipolar disorder. It may also sometimes be used in conjunction with antidepressants to treat depression. Lithium has properties similar to sodium and potassium and interferes with the action of sodium in neuromuscular cells, reducing agitation. It also interferes with the production and action of neurotransmitters and affects levels of tryptophan and serotonin in the central nervous system. It can also cause an increase in leukocyte production. Lithium crosses the placenta so it should not be taken during pregnancy or while nursing. Overdosing can cause severe side effects so blood levels must be routinely monitored. Side effects include hand tremors, twitching, nausea, diarrhea, seizures, confusion, and increase in urinary output. About 1 patient in 25 develops goiter from lithium-induced hypothyroidism. Non-steroidal anti-inflammatory drugs (NSAIDs), selective serotonin reuptake inhibitors (SSRIs), phenothiazines, and diuretics may cause drug interactions.

Work-up required before starting lithium
Lithium has a very narrow therapeutic window, and toxicity is a medical emergency that can lead to death. Lithium is cleared from the body by the kidneys and can negatively affect thyroid function. An initial assessment should include an evaluation of kidney function. Tests include a urinalysis (UA), blood urea nitrogen (BUN) and creatinine levels, an electrolyte panel, 24-hour urine for creatinine clearance, screening for diabetes, hypertension, and any history of diuretic medications or over use of analgesics. Thyroid function must also be evaluated. A TSH, T3, T4 and free thyroxine index should be drawn. A complete physical exam along with a complete family and patient history should be obtained. Other tests should include a 12-lead electrocardiogram (ECG), fasting blood glucose, and complete blood count (CBC).

Depakote®

Divalproex (Depakote®), a derivative of valproic acid, has the fewest side effects, adverse reactions, and lowest potential for toxicity of all anticonvulsants used to treat bipolar disorder. This medication has become the first-line medication choice for treatment of bipolar disorder because of its low potential for toxicity and effective treatment in several subgroups of bipolar disorder. It is usually well tolerated by the patient with side effects including gastrointestinal upset, tremors, drowsiness, headache, vertigo, and ataxia. It has also been associated with increased appetite and weight gain. The appearance of unexplained bruising, petechiae, or bleeding can indicate thrombocytopenia and the drug must be stopped. The most dangerous adverse side effect to this medication is severe liver damage. Liver function tests are obtained before starting the drug, then every 1-4 weeks for 6 months, followed by routine evaluations every 3-6 months throughout treatment. This medication is contraindicated during pregnancy.

Carbamazepine

Carbamazepine (Tegretol®) is considered a third-line medication choice for bipolar disorder. Divalproex and lithium are usually used in treatment before this medication choice. This medication can be added for use in combination medication therapy. Side effects can include sleepiness, vertigo, ataxia, blurred or double vision, gastrointestinal upset, fatigue, or, in rare cases, rash. Carbamazepine is metabolized by the cytochrome (CYP)-450 enzyme found in the liver and can lead to dangerous interactions and decreased effectiveness of other anticonvulsants, anticoagulants (such as warfarin), or oral birth control pills. Carbamazepine can lead to agranulocytosis, which is a decrease in the white blood cell count that can lead to fatal infections.

Benzodiazepines

Benzodiazepines are the most commonly prescribed medications for anxiety. Some of the more commonly prescribed include chlordiazepoxide, lorazepam, diazepam, flurazepam, and triazolam. Benzodiazepines act to enhance the neurotransmitter gamma-aminobutyric acid (GABA). This neurotransmitter inhibits the firing rate of neurons and therefore leads to a decline in anxiety symptoms. Indications for their use can include anxiety, insomnia disorders, alcohol withdrawal, seizure control, skeletal muscle relation, or agitation. They can also be utilized to reduce the anxiety symptoms pre-operatively or before any other type of medical procedure such as cardiac catheterization or colonoscopy. This class of drug is also the treatment of choice for alcohol withdrawal. Benzodiazepines are used to treat insomnia because of their sedative-hypnotic effects. When using a sedative-hypnotic to treat sleep disturbances, the medication should have rapid onset and allow the patient to wake up feeling refreshed instead of tired and groggy. When administered at bedtime, most benzodiazepines will produce a sleep-inducing effect and should be used on a short-term basis.

Buspirone

Due to the addictive potential of benzodiazepines, the use of non-benzodiazepines to treat anxiety has increased. One of the most commonly used non-benzodiazepines is buspirone. This medication is highly effective in treating anxiety and its associated symptoms, such as insomnia, poor concentration, tension, restlessness, irritability, and fatigue. Buspirone had no addictive potential, is not useful in alcohol withdrawal or seizures or known to interact with other central nervous system depressants. Because it may take several weeks of continual use for the effects of this drug to be realized by the patient, it cannot be used on an as needed basis. Buspirone does not increase depression symptoms and therefore is useful in treating anxiety associated with depression. Side effects associated with medication can include gastrointestinal upset, dizziness, sleepiness, excitement, or headache.

First-generation antipsychotics

There are a variety of first-generation antipsychotics available, though their use is becoming less prominent now that atypical antipsychotic agents are available. Some first-generation antipsychotics include: chlorpromazine (Thorazine®), thioridazine hydrochloride (Mellaril®), haloperidol (Haldol®), pimozide (Orap®), fluphenazine hydrochloride (Prolixin®), molindone hydrochloride (Moban®), and trifluoperazine hydrochloride (Stelazine®). Possible side effects include: photosensitivity, sexual dysfunction, dry mouth, dry eyes, nasal congestion, blurred vision, constipation, urinary retention, exacerbation of narrow-angle glaucoma, various cardiac effects, extrapyramidal effects, dyskinesia, sedation, cognitive dulling, amenorrhea, menstrual irregularities, hyperglycemia or hypoglycemia, increased appetite, and weight gain. Drug interactions depend on the individual drug.

Second-generation/atypical antipsychotics

Second-generation antipsychotics (SGAs), also called atypical antipsychotics, are used for bipolar disorders, schizophrenia, and psychosis and include aripiprazole (Abilify®), clozapine (Clozaril®), olanzapine (Zyprexa®), quetiapine (Seroquel®), risperidone (Risperdal®), and ziprasidone (Geodon®). Females report more side effects than males, but the recommended doses for males and females are identical. Women were underrepresented when SGAs were clinically tested because researchers feared teratogenic effects on fetuses. Side effects include constipation, increased appetite, weight gain, urinary retention, various sexual side effects, increased prolactin, menstrual irregularities, increased risk of diabetes mellitus, decreased blood pressure, dizziness, agranulocytosis, and leucopenia. Atypical antipsychotics may interact with fluvoxamine, phenytoin, carbamazepine, barbiturates, nicotine, ketoconazole, phenytoin, rifampin, and glucocorticoids. The use of atypical antipsychotic agents correlates with significant weight gain. Overweight and obese patients are likely to develop insulin resistance and glucose intolerance, which may lead to diabetes mellitus. Data show clozapine and olanzapine as the greatest offenders. Ziprasidone seems to present the lowest risk.

Melatonin

Melatonin is a natural hormone that serves to regulate sleep and circadian rhythms. This dietary supplement has been investigated as a therapy and/or adjunct therapy for treating seasonal affective disorder (SAD), bipolar disorder, attention-deficit hyperactivity, jet lag, sleep disorders, and solid tumor cancers as well as for learning and memory enhancement. The dose for all but cancer is sublingual, 2.5 mg to 3.0 mg at bedtime only. The dose for cancer is 20 mg with chemotherapy. Melatonin is not regulated by the Food and Drug Administration (FDA). Therefore, all use of melatonin should be monitored closely, especially when it is used in conjunction with psychotropic medications. Melatonin is generally well tolerated. The only apparent side effects are potentiation of the effects of sedatives and mild headaches.

Serotonin syndrome, baclofen withdrawal, and benzodiazepine withdrawal

- Serotonin syndrome: This life-threatening reaction usually results from taking an overdose of medication that causes levels of serotonin to increase or combining two medications, such as an SSRI with a triptan. Drugs that contribute include antidepressants, opioids, psychedelics, St. John's wort, lithium, and CNS stimulants. Effects include cognitive (confusion, hallucinations), autonomic (tachycardia, nausea, diarrhea, hyperthermia), and somatic (myoclonus, tremor, hyperreflexia). Treatment includes stopping drugs, administering antagonist (cyproheptadine), and providing supportive interventions.
- Baclofen withdrawal: Baclofen is a central-acting muscle relaxant used for treatment of muscle spasticity. Patients may experience withdrawal symptoms when the medication is discontinued, especially after more than two to three months of use. Symptoms are worse with abrupt discontinuation and abate with readministration. Symptoms include hallucinations, delusions, confusion, nausea, autonomic dysfunction, fever, muscle rigidity, memory impairment, and seizures.
- Benzodiazepine withdrawal: Benzodiazepines are depressants used to relieve anxiety. Abrupt withdrawal after prolonged use may result in autonomic withdrawal symptoms (similar to baclofen) with increased agitation, muscular weakness, seizures, tremors, hypertension, and tachycardia. Treatment includes tapering of drug dosage and administration of diazepam.

Steroid-induced psychosis and antibiotic-induced mania

- Steroid-induced psychosis occurs in about 5-6% of patients receiving steroids with higher doses (at least 40 mg prednisone or equivalent) most likely to result in symptoms. Onset, usually preceded by state of hyperexcitability, is with six to ten hours for parenteral drugs and four to 6 days for oral. Symptoms vary widely with about 40% primarily depressive but some exhibit mania, delirium and paranoid psychosis. Incidence is highest in females and most common with lupus erythematosus (about 40%) and pemphigus (about 20%).

- Antibiotic-induced mania (AKA antibiomania) is a rare onset of acute mania, which may include psychosis and paranoia, associated with administration of antibiotics. In the United States, the drugs most commonly associated with the disorder are clarithromycin and ciprofloxacin, but a wide range of other antibiotics, including isoniazid and penicillin, have been implicated. Discontinuing the medication should result in resolution of the symptoms.

Common interactions

Prozac
Prozac® (fluoxetine hydrochloride) is an SSRI antidepressant that is indicated for treatment of depression, OCD, bulimia nervosa, panic disorder, PTSD, premenstrual dysphoric disorder, and depressive disorders associated with bipolar I disorder. Prozac has many interactions that the nurse practitioner must be aware of when prescribing Prozac.

- Drug-drug interactions: Because of multiple drug-drug interactions, when prescribing Prozac®, the nurse practitioner should always check the list of interactions against the patient's list of drugs. Drug-drug interactions that increase risk of serotonin syndrome include MAO inhibitors (avoid use of Prozac within 5 weeks), amphetamines, tricyclic antidepressants, tramadol, and other SSRIs and SSNRIs. Drugs that increase CNS effects include benzodiazepine, lithium, and tricyclic antidepressants. Prozac® may potentiate the effects of beta-blockers, carbamazepine, flecainide, and vinblastine. Prozac® may alter glucose levels when used with insulin and oral antidiabetics, so dosage of these drugs may need to be adjusted.
- Drug-herb interactions: Serotonin syndrome may occur with St. John's wort. Patients may experience increased sedative effect with the two drugs.
- Drug-lifestyle interactions: Alcohol may increase CNS depression and should not be used with Prozac®.

Psychiatric medications and Theophylline
Theophylline is a methylxanthine used to treat bronchospasm, but it must be used with care with some psychiatric medications. Interactions include:

- Lithium: Theophylline increases the rate of renal clearance of lithium, so the dosage of lithium must be increased in order to maintain the appropriate serum level, usually by about 60%; however, because of the narrow therapeutic range of lithium, dosage should be titrated carefully and serum levels monitored frequently.
- Benzodiazepines (diazepam, lorazepam, flurazepam): Theophylline blocks adenosine receptors while benzodiazepines increase CNS concentration of adenosine. This results in the need for greater diazepam dosage to reach the desired effects. Because of the increased dosage, if the theophylline is discontinued, patients may experience respiratory depression.
- St. John's wort: This herbal drug decreases the concentration of theophylline in the plasma, so if the St. John's wort is discontinued, the patient may experience theophylline toxicity.

Lithium toxicity

Plasma levels of lithium must be frequently monitored for lithium toxicity, which can lead to death. The normal therapeutic range is 0.6 and 1.4 mEq/L for adults. Plasma levels will usually decrease to an acceptable level within 48 hours after discontinuation of the medication; however, in severe cases involving acute renal failure, dialysis may be necessary. A complete initial assessment, ongoing assessments, frequent evaluations of lithium levels, and patient education are all an essential part of the treatment plan. A patient must be able to tell the difference between side effects and symptoms of toxicity. Symptoms of mild toxicity associated with blood levels between 1.5–2.5 mEq/L can include severe vomiting and diarrhea, increased muscle tremors and twitching, lethargy, body aches, ataxia, ringing in the ears, blurry vision, vertigo, or hyperactive deep tendon reflexes. More severe symptoms associated with blood levels >2.5 mEq/L can include elevated temperature, low urine output, hypotension, electrocardiogram (ECG) abnormalities, decreased level of consciousness, seizures, coma, or death.

Benzodiazepine toxicity

Benzodiazepine toxicity may result from accidental or intentional overdose with such drugs as Xanax®, Librium®, Valium®, Ativan®, Serax®, Versed®, and Restoril®. Mortality is usually the result of co-ingestion of other drugs. Symptoms are often non-specific neurological changes: lethargy, dizziness, alterations in consciousness, and ataxia. Respiratory depression and hypotension are rare complications. Coma and severe central nervous depression is usually is caused by co-ingestions. Diagnosis is based on history and clinical exam, as benzodiazepine level does not correlate well with toxicity. Treatment includes:
- Gastric emptying (<1 hour).
- Charcoal.
- Concentrated dextrose, thiamine, and naloxone if co-ingestions suspected, especially with altered mental status.
- Monitoring for central nervous system/respiratory depression.
- Supportive care.
- Flumazenil (antagonist) 0.2 mg each minute to total 3 mg may be used in some cases but not routinely advised because of complications related to benzodiazepine dependency or co-ingestion of cyclic antidepressants. Flumazenil is contraindicated in the presence of increased intracranial pressure.

Extrapyramidal effects of first-generation antipsychotics and neuroleptics

The extrapyramidal system is a group of neural connections outside of the medulla that control movement. Extrapyramidal effects are the result of drug influence on the extrapyramidal system and include:
- Akinesia (inability to start movement).
- Akathisia (inability to stop movement).
- Dystonia (extreme and uncontrolled muscle contraction, torticollis, flexing, and twisting).

The most common extrapyramidal symptom caused by antipsychotic agents is tardive dyskinesia, in which patients are unable to control their movements, such as tics, lip smacking, and eye blinking. The term tardive refers to the delayed onset of the symptoms. Even after the discontinuation of a drug, extrapyramidal side effects may still be present. Oculogyric crisis is common in children, and features restlessness, staring, painful deviation or crossing of the eyes, jaw spasm, and protruding tongue. Antipsychotics also cause Parkinsonian symptoms like lead-pipe muscle rigidity, but these symptoms occur most often in elderly adults.

Neuroleptic malignant syndrome

Neuroleptic malignant syndrome (NMS) is 1 of the most serious complicating side effects associated with use of antipsychotic medications. Initiating antipsychotics, haloperidol, benzamines, tricyclics, monoamine oxidase (MAO) inhibitors, and lithium too fast can cause NMS. This potentially fatal and rare condition can result with 1 single dosage of medication. The highest risk medications fall into the high-potency category. Symptoms occur acutely and can include high fever, tachycardia, diaphoresis, rigid muscles, shaking, incontinence, confusion and decreased level of consciousness, renal failure, and elevated creatine phosphokinase (CPK) levels. It is very important to always monitor a patient's temperature with use of antipsychotics. The patient may require supportive care in the form of resuscitation, mechanical ventilation, hydration, and fever reducing actions. All antipsychotic drugs must be discontinued and the patient may be treated with dantrolene or bromocriptine. Development of this side effect does not exclude the patient from future treatment with antipsychotic medications.

Treatment for extrapyramidal effects

Extrapyramidal effects drastically alter a patient's quality of life by making him/her conspicuous in public. The patient can also develop frightening dysphagia (difficulty swallowing) and depression. One must treat the symptoms in order to maintain an effective psychopharmacological therapy or risk the patient's discontinuation of the drugs due to their motor side effects. Symptom control agents of choice include:
- Anticholinergics, such as benztropine or biperiden.
- Antiviral amantadine hydrochloride, which mediate symptoms by increasing dopamine activity in the brain.
- Bromocriptine.
- Pergolide.

Adult studies have shown that vitamin E may mediate extrapyramidal symptoms, though research regarding pediatric use is limited.

Tardive dyskinesia

Tardive dyskinesia (TD) is a chronic syndrome that can develop as a result of the long-term use of antipsychotic medications. The elderly population is at the highest risk for development of this syndrome. There is currently no effective treatment and the best defense is early detection and prevention of symptoms. Use of the lowest effective dosage of an atypical antipsychotic is often recommended for prevention. TDs are abnormal movements of the tongue, lips, face, trunk, and extremities. Patients with schizophrenia appear especially vulnerable to developing TDs after exposure to neuroleptics, anticholinergics, toxins, and substances of abuse. If caused by medication, TDs continue in 50% of patients even if the medication is stopped. Symptoms include:
- Lip smacking or puckering.
- Tongue protrusion.
- Eyelid blinking.
- Repetitive tapping.
- Marching movement.
- Choreiform movements of the extremities and trunk.
- Occasional spasm of diaphragm or muscles involved in swallowing which can lead to choking or respiratory problems.

Polypharmacy

Mental health patients are at risk for polypharmacy, taking too many drugs, because of taking the same drug under generic and brand names, taking drugs for 1 condition but contraindicated for another, and taking drugs that are not compatible. Reasons for polypharmacy include multiple prescriptions from different doctors; forgetfulness; confusion; failure to report current medications; the use of supplemental, over-the-counter, and herbal preparations in addition to prescribed medications; and failure of healthcare providers to adequately educate the patient. Patients should be encouraged to keep a list of all current medications (prescribed and otherwise) and to bring all medications with him/her to appointments. If family members are present, they should be enlisted in ensuring the patient avoids polypharmacy. Healthcare providers must take the time to discuss medications with the patient to ensure that the patient understands and must ask directly if the patient is taking any other medications. Helping the patient to make lifestyle changes, such as dieting or quitting smoking, may reduce the need for medications.

Hyponatremia and hypoglycemia in patients being evaluated for acute psychosis

The clinical significance of hyponatremia and hypoglycemia in the patient being evaluated for acute psychosis:
- Hyponatremia: While severe hyponatremia may occur without psychiatric illness, it is not uncommon in psychiatric patients and may relate to worsening symptoms of disease, water intoxication related to compulsive polydipsia, compulsive smoking/drinking, and drug abuse. Additionally, some antipsychotic agents and antidepressants are associated with hyponatremia. Signs and symptoms include not only acute psychosis but also alterations in consciousness, hallucinations, tremor, seizures, impaired cognition, coma, and life-threatening electrolyte imbalance.
- Hypoglycemia: While the classic signs of hypoglycemia include tremor, tachycardia, weakness, anxiety, and hunger, hypoglycemia may manifest with a wide variety of symptoms affecting multiple body systems, sometimes making diagnosis difficult. Because the central nervous system depends on carbohydrates for fuel, when the blood glucose level drops, one of the first indications is neurologic dysfunction, usually resulting in alterations of consciousness. Patients may be confused, lethargic, combative and/or extremely agitated. Sensorium may be depressed, and some patients develop seizures and focal neurologic deficits. Symptoms generally reverse promptly with administration of glucose.

Hypoxemia per ABG in patients being evaluated for acute psychosis

The normal value of PaO2 is 80 to 100 mm Hg and SaO2 is 96 to 98%. Hypoxemia occurs when the level of oxygen in the arterial system falls below 80 mm Hg. This in turn may result in *hypoxia*, a lack of adequate oxygenation at the tissue level. The brain is particularly susceptible to hypoxia with impaired functioning of the cerebral tissue within one minute of onset of hypoxia. The severity of neuropsychiatric symptoms relates to the rate and degree of hypoxic onset. Patients may tolerate a slow onset with minimal symptoms even at 60 mm Hg; but, if hypoxia occurs abruptly, the patient may have a concomitant abrupt onset of acute psychosis and delirium. Even mild hypoxia may produce changes in cognition with the patient having difficulty using language and understanding abstractions as well as coordinating motor activity. Patients may be extremely drowsy or emotionally labile. If hypoxia is severe, the patient may lose consciousness and/or experience seizures.

Ruling out drug toxicities and overdoses while evaluating the patient

When evaluating the patient, the nurse practitioner must often rule out drug toxicities and overdoses when determining the diagnosis. Toxic reactions to drugs and overdoses can mimic other mental health disorders. Methods include:
- Screening: Various screening tests are available to screen for a wide variety of drugs (amphetamines, barbiturates, marijuana, cocaine, PCP, methadone, benzodiazepines, and barbiturates) and alcohol. Blood, urine, and sputum tests may be ordered.
- Physical examination: The nurse should be aware of physical and other signs of substance abuse, such as needle tracks, fingertip burns, dilated or constricted pupils, repeated sniffing, tremors, odor of marijuana/alcohol, and lack of personal hygiene. Patients may exhibit labile mood swings and impulsive or inappropriate behavior. Overdose is often associated with excess sedation and somnolence leading to coma.
- History: A careful history and review of previous medical records may provide information about drug use. If asked, patients may admit to using drugs, so the direct approach may be useful.

Depression and aging/co-morbid conditions

Depression affects about 19% of adults >55 and 37% of older adults with co-morbid conditions, putting older adults (who have the highest rates of suicide) at risk. Depression is associated with conditions that decrease quality of life, such as heart disease, neuromuscular diseases, arthritis, cancer, diabetes, Huntington's disease, stroke, and diabetes. Some drugs may also precipitate depression: diuretics, Parkinson's drugs, estrogen, corticosteroids, cimetidine, hydralazine, Propranolol, digitalis, and indomethacin. Patients experience changes in mood, sadness, loss of interest in usual activities, increased fatigue, changes in appetite and fluctuations in weight, anxiety, and sleep disturbance. Depression often goes undiagnosed, so screening for at-risk individuals should be done routinely. Treatment includes tricyclic antidepressants (TCAs) and selective serotonin reuptake inhibitors (SSRIs), but SSRIs have fewer side effects and are less likely to cause death with an overdose. Older adults may take longer to respond to medication than younger adults. Counselling, treating underlying cause, and instituting an exercise program may help reduce depression.

Genetics and mental illness

Genetic inheritance has a profound effect on the development of some mental illness, especially schizophrenia and depression. Most psychiatric disorders are caused by a combination of factors, such as genetic makeup, peripartum stressors and influences, environmental influences, and family and social stressors. Eliciting family history of mental illness is a very important aspect of case management as it may bring to light genetic predisposition for illness, particularly if a first-degree relative has a disorder. An individual may have a high level of genetic risk if mental illness is prevalent in the family, or a low level of genetic risk if it is absent. If genetic risk is present, that individual is much more susceptible to developing mental illness as he/she ages, experiences life stressors, or is negatively influenced by environmental interactions.

Heritability
Heritability is the genetic contribution to phenotype in a specific population of individuals. This genetic contribution is affected by maternal and paternal genetic contributions and allelic and dominance variations. Heritability may be estimated by statistical means that take into account both genetic and environmental variances on a given population. Heritability may be estimated

using regression and correlation models (comparison of close relatives, siblings, twins, parents, and offspring) or analysis of variance (equations and coefficients of variance). Because mental illness is often directly correlated with genetic predisposition, predicted heritability patterns may expose a genetic predisposition for illness, such as schizophrenia or chronic depression, before symptoms present. In some cases, patients may express concern about their offspring inheriting mental illness. Research indicates that genetic variations can markedly increase risk of developing mental illness in relation to stress and other environmental issues.

Functional neurological symptoms

Functional neurological symptoms relate to impaired function of the neurological system that is unrelated to diagnostic evidence of damage to the neurological system and may encompass a wide range of symptoms, including limb weakness, tremors, dystonia, slurred speech, dysphagia, anxiety, poor concentration/memory, pain, sleep problems, and excessive fatigue. For example, with limb weakness, mobility and strength may be impaired, but reflexes remain intact and testing (CT, MRI) shows no abnormalities. Additionally, if the contralateral limb is exercised or stressed, the symptoms often disappear temporarily. In fact, symptoms often vary in intensity. The cause of functional neurological symptoms may be difficult to pinpoint although sometimes they occur after injury or illness, but functional neurological symptoms generally relate to impairment of transmission of impulses in the nervous system. While some symptoms may be related to malingering or psychiatric disease, in most cases this is not true although that is a common misperception. Treatment approaches vary depending on the type of symptoms.

Assessment components

Upon a patient's admission to care, the assessment components include:
- Presenting symptoms: The nurse should note the general appearance and the type of symptoms, including abnormal motor behavior such as automatisms, psychomotor retardation, and waxy flexibility as well as posture and eye contact.
- Degree of thought organization: The nurse should evaluate both thought content and thought processes and note circumstantial thinking; delusions; flight of ideas; loose associations; tangential thinking; thought blocking; broadcasting; insertion; withdrawal; word salad; and ideas of reference.
- Mood and affect: Mood is the patients underlying emotional state while affect is the outward expression of that state. Mood may be characterized as happy, sad, angry, or anxious. Mood swings (labile mood) should be noted as well as inconsistencies between mood and affect or mood and situation. Affect is categorized as blunted (showing little expression), broad (showing a broad range of expressions), flat (showing no expression), inappropriate (expression does not match mood or situation), and restricted (showing only one type of expression).
- Hygiene: The nurse should note the condition of the patient's skin, nails, teeth, and hair and whether the patient is clean or needs bathing. The nurse may note signs of lice, such as scratching or nits, and whether clothes are clean or soiled.
- Grooming: The patient's grooming should include whether the patient appears unkempt. Is the hair combed and patient shaved? Completely or partially dressed? Are clothes appropriate?

- Short/Long term memory: The nurse should ask questions that probe both short-term memory, "What did you have for lunch?" and long-term "Who was the president before the current one?" Additionally, questions should probe general orientation: "What state is this?" "What is your social security number?" "What is your home address?" The nurse should also assess concentration, such as by asking the patient to repeat a list of numbers backward or perform a three-part task. Assessing abstract thinking can include asking the patient to interpret a common proverb to determine if the patient understands the meaning.

Neuropsychological tests

Neuropsychological tests assess the effects of brain damage or impairment on intellectual, motor, and/or emotional functioning. In adults, impairment may be related to various causes while in children it usually relates to congenital or perinatal conditions. Testing results may help to identify the cause for cognitive deficits and may provide information about the areas of the brain damaged and the extent of injury. In children, it may identify the cause of educational delays and learning disabilities. Patients may undergo fixed batteries of tests or individual tests. A number of different tests are used depending on the function to be evaluated: intelligence (general and premorbid), language (general and comprehension), memory, attention, visuospatial ability, apraxia, reasoning, and handedness. The most commonly utilized tests are the Wechsler Adult Intelligence Scales (WAIS, WAIS-R, and WAIS-III). WAIS-III, the current version, comprises 14 subtests and two major scales (verbal IQ and performance IQ). Other tests include the Stanford-Binet Intelligence Scale, the Halstead-Reitan Battery, and the Luria-Nebraska Neuropsychological Battery. A pediatric version of WAIS-III is available. Another pediatric assessment is the Rivermead Behavioural Memory Test.

EEG testing in patient with altered level of consciousness

The electroencephalogram is sometimes used to test patients with altered level of consciousness in order to evaluate the patients' electrical impulses (brain waves). EEG is indicated for suspected seizure activity, encephalopathies, infarcts, and altered consciousness. The purpose is to identify abnormal electrical activity, which may be noted as slowing, which occurs where there has been injury or an infarct. Waves include delta (1-4 cycles/sec), alpha (8-13 cycles/sec), theta (4-7 cycles/sec), beta (12-40 cycles/sec), sleep spindles (12-14 cycles/sec), and spikes and waves (variable duration). Spikes and waves indicate that tissue is irritated. Findings indicate:
- Metabolic encephalopathy: Intermittent slowing with triphasic waves.
- Cerebral anoxic damage: Generalized slowing in delta and theta range.
- Coma state: Prognosis poor if EEG showing unchanging alpha waves with stimulation.
- CNS depressant overdose: Transient periods of absence of electrical activity.
- Epilepsy: Unusual electrical activity within the brain. Partial seizures are evident in only part of the electrodes while generalized seizures are evident from all electrodes.
- ADHD: a 20-minute EEG procedure is FDA-approved to diagnose children with ADHD.

Appropriate testing for patient presenting with delirium

Appropriate testing for a patient presenting with delirium, transient confusion and alterations in consciousness, depends on the age and circumstances. Delirium is most common in older adults in response to illness or surgery but can occur at any age. Hyperactive delirium may be associated with alcohol withdrawal or drug toxicity. Hypoactive delirium may result from disease processes, such as hepatic encephalopathy. Some have mixed symptoms, becoming more agitated during the evening and night.

Testing includes:

- Confusion Assessment Method (CAM) or CAM-ICU: This test helps to differentiate confusion from other causes of altered consciousness.
- CAM-S: This form of the CAM test is used to determine the severity of delirium.
- Delirium Symptom Interview also helps to identify delirium.
- Laboratory tests: If the cause of the patient's confusion is not evident, numerous tests may be done to rule out other causes, including CBC, blood glucose, renal and liver function tests, drug and alcohol screening, sed-rate, thyroid function tests, HIV, and thiamine and vitamin B-12 levels.

Laboratory tests for patients presenting with new onset psychiatric issue

When patients present with a new onset psychiatric issue, a series of laboratory tests may be conducted to determine potential causes, rule out differential diagnoses, and identify concomitant disorders:

- Blood alcohol level and urine drug screening to determine if the patient is experiencing overdosing, withdrawal symptoms, or toxic reaction.
- Blood glucose level to determine if the patient has hypoglycemia or hyperglycemia that may be affecting mental status.
- Urinalysis and urine culture to determine if an infection is present (may result in confusion in older adults).
- Brain imaging (CT, MRI) to determine if a lesion is present in the brain.
- Pregnancy testing to determine if female patients are pregnant before initiating treatment.
- Liver and kidney function tests to evaluate for hepatic and renal encephalopathy.
- CBC to assess for anemia, infection, or other abnormalities.
- HIV antibodies to rule out HIV/AIDS.
- EEG to determine if the patient is experiencing seizure activity.
- Lyme antibodies to rule out neuropsychological symptoms related to Lyme disease.
- Lumbar puncture to examine cerebrospinal fluid for suspected infection.

Utility of laboratory tests for psychiatric illnesses

At the current time, diagnosis of psychiatric illnesses is based almost completely on symptoms and history, and no laboratory tests have been FDA approved for diagnosis; however, biochemical markers have been identified for some psychiatric disorders, including schizophrenia, bipolar disorder, and depression. Some companies have collected data and applied for FDA approval for these tests and are now marketing tests although this testing is not in common use because use is not yet reimbursed by Medicare/Medicaid or insurance companies. Some researchers believe that genetic testing and imaging (PET, MRI) may also have larger roles in diagnosis in the future. Currently, laboratory tests are used for primarily two reasons:

- Rule out differential diagnoses and identify concomitant disorders. Many different tests may be used, but in many cases the results of tests don't alter the original diagnosis, so testing is done selectively, based on patient's age, history, and physical exam.
- Monitor serum levels of drugs during therapy, such as lithium levels.

Interpreting results of head CT for patient with altered mental status

The CT scan is a common imaging technique used to diagnose patients who present with altered mental status. The CT scan can identify traumatic brain injury and mass lesions, such as brain tumors or hematomas, as well as cerebral edema, so it may be invaluable for neurological disorders, but it is primarily used to rule out differential diagnoses rather than to diagnose mental health disorders. CT scans may also be used in addition to other tests to help confirm a possible diagnosis. For example, patients with schizophrenia tend to have enlarged ventricles with increased CSF and a concomitant reduction in brain volume with sulci that are more widened than in a non-schizophrenic brain. Despite these findings, the CT alone cannot be used for diagnosis, and no specific pattern of abnormality has been noted with depression or bipolar disorder although there is evidence that the frontal cortex shrinks in size with uncontrolled bipolar disease and depression and increases with treatment, so long-term monitoring may show differences.

Hypercalcemia

Hypercalcemia is an elevated serum calcium level. There are numerous causes; the most common are hypoparathyroidism and cancer. Clinical manifestations of hypercalcemia include fatigue, weakness, confusion, passage of renal stones, nausea, vomiting and abdominal pain. The diagnosis is made by laboratory examination of serum calcium, parathyroid hormone (PTH) and phosphate levels. Order CT scan or chest x-ray to rule out malignancy. The goal of treatment is to lower the calcium level. Possible treatments include IV fluids, calcitonin, corticosteroids, IV bisphosphonates, oral phosphate, and dialysis as a last resort. Primary hyperparathyroidism can be treated surgically. Underlying malignancy should be treated appropriately.

Prevalence of disorders

Mood disorders
Depression onset varies but is most common in young adulthood (mid-20s) and the recurrence rate is about 60%.
Bipolar disorders:
- Bipolar I disorder occurs in up to 1.6% adults, with onset usually in early adulthood, although older psychiatric patients have higher rates of about 20%.
- Bipolar II disorder is less common, occurring in about 0.5% of the population, and occurs more frequently in females than males.
- Cyclothymic disorder occurs in 0.4 to 1% with onset in adolescence or early adulthood.

Psychotic disorders
Schizophrenia occurs in up to 1.5% of adults with onset usually in early adulthood (20s). Those with first-degree family members with the disease have a risk of developing schizophrenia 10 times higher than the general public. Schizoaffective disorder usually begins in early adulthood, more commonly in females than males, and affects <1% of the population, although these patients are at high risk for substance abuse and suicide.
Delusional disorders affect only about 0.3% of the population, with onset usually in adolescence or later, with incidence increasing to 2 to 4% in older adults. Shared psychotic disorder (Folie a deux) is rare (prevalence unclear) but appears to affect females more than males. Age of onset varies widely.

Dissociative disorders

Dissociative amnesia is an area of controversy. Prevalence is unknown but reported cases are rising, although some researchers believe it is over-diagnosed in people who are suggestible. Dissociative identity disorder (multiple personality) is an area of controversy as some people experiencing dissociative identity disorders are responding to suggestions. Prevalence is not clear but dissociative identity disorder is more common in females than males. Dissociative fugue occurs rarely, affecting only about 0.2% of the general population although increased rates may occur in times of severe stress, such as during war or natural disasters. Depersonalization disorder may occur in about half the population in response to stress, but statistics are not available. However, depersonalization is observed in about 40% of hospitalized psychiatric patients.

Anxiety disorders

Phobias of all types are fairly common in the general population, affecting between 7.2 and 11.3% of the population over a lifetime, with rates decreasing with age. Obsessive-compulsive disorder occurs in up to 2.3% of adults, with rates higher in those whose first-degree family members have the same disorder. Post-traumatic stress syndrome ranges from 1 to 14% in the general population over the course of a lifetime, but at-risk populations, such as those that have experienced abuse, have much higher rates, ranging from 3 to 64%. Incidence is about twice as high in females as in males, often associated with physical, emotional, or sexual abuse. Generalized anxiety disorder (GAD) occurs in up to 5% of the adult population with about two-thirds of people with GAD being female. Panic disorder affects up to 2% of the population but about 10% of those referred for psychiatric evaluation. Panic disorder is often associated with agoraphobia.

Sleep disorders

Insomnia is a common problem occurring in up to 35% of adults at some time in their life, with chronic insomnia occurring in 10 to 15% of adults. Insomnia may be precipitated by physical conditions, such as heart disease, gastroesophageal reflux disease (GERD), urinary incontinence, or psychiatric disorders. Insomnia is common with depression and bipolar disorder. Narcolepsy is a rare disorder occurring in only 0.02 to 0.16% of adults, with onset usually occurring in adolescence (although symptoms may be evident earlier). Breathing-related sleep disorders affect up to 10% of the population, with increased incidence in older adults. Onset of symptoms is usually between ages 40 and 60. Circadian Rhythm Sleep Disorder, common among shift workers, occurs in up to 4% of adults and 7% of adolescents, with onset typically during adolescence and often proceeded by an episode of stress.

Eating disorders/substance abuse

Anorexia nervosa is 10 times more common in females than males and affects about 0.5 to 1% of the population. Onset is usually during adolescence between ages 14 and 16. Bulimia nervosa affects between 3 and 8% of the population, with onset in the late teens or early adulthood between ages 18 and 24. Like anorexia, bulimia is 10 times more common in females than males. Alcoholism affects about 16% of the population with about 20% of those over age 12 engaging in periodic binge drinking. Illicit drugs are used by about 6.3% of the population over age 12, with marijuana being the most commonly used illicit drug.

Personality disorders

Borderline personality disorder affects 2 to 20% of the general population but up to 20% of hospitalized psychiatric patients. The disorder becomes evident during adolescence, but symptoms often lessen with age. Schizotypal personality disorder affects about 3% of the general population with a higher rate (about 17%) in diagnosed psychiatric patients.

Antisocial personality disorder occurs in about 3.6% of the adult population with males at higher risk for the disorder than females and onset during childhood. Paranoid personality disorder affects up to 2.5% of the general population but up to 30% of those hospitalized for psychiatric disorders.

Correctional institutions and mental illness

The Bureau of Justice Statistics estimates that about 16% of inmates in adult prisons and jails suffer from mental illness. Correctional institutions are often severely overcrowded and lack resources to adequately care for patients. The increasing rate of mentally ill inmates may relate to deinstitutionalization that resulted in large numbers of mentally ill people becoming homeless with some becoming involved in substance abuse and criminal activity. In most correctional facilities, the mentally ill are housed with the general population, leaving them vulnerable to abuse. Mentally ill inmates, such as those with schizophrenia, may find it difficult or impossible to follow rules, so they may be punished for misconduct with loss of privileges, solitary confinement, or extended sentence, all increasing anxiety and stress. Treatment, if available, is often geared toward controlling behavior rather than treating the disorder.

Homeless population

The homeless population has disproportionate rates of mental illness, estimated at about 40 to 45%, many with serious illnesses, such as schizophrenia and bipolar disorder, complicated by substance abuse. The need for adequate housing is an ongoing problem with homeless patients. Once released from inpatient care services, the homeless do not have anywhere to live. A safe and affordable option is vital to the success of their treatment. Many of these patients have a relapse of their mental illnesses, suffer medical illnesses, incarceration, or abuse by others. The homeless often resist treatment (sometimes not believing they are ill), fail to keep appointments, and lack transportation or money for transportation. They may have no money for medications, may not qualify for assistance, or may be reluctant to deal with government agencies in order to gain assistance.

Mental illness among migrant workers

Migrant workers are at risk for mental illness because of long hours, stress about providing for families, and using substance abuse as a coping mechanism. Many are non-English speakers, undocumented, far from family support systems, experiencing racism, and lacking access to medical care. Mental health issues of primary concern for migrant workers are depression, stress, substance abuse, and domestic violence. Most migrant workers are ethnic minorities, and some feel a stigma is attached to mental health problems and may resist treatment even if outreach programs are available or may fear loss of employment if they get treatment. Additionally, they may lack transportation to get to treatment or a flexible schedule to allow them to keep appointments. Programs for migrant workers must be affordable and should address both language and cultural concerns and allow for flexible hours to accommodate work schedules.

Therapeutic communication

Therapeutic communication begins with respect for the patient/family and the assumption that all communication, verbal and non-verbal, has meaning. Listening must be done empathetically. Techniques that facilitate communication include:

Introduction	Make a personal introduction and use the patient's name: "Mrs. Brown, I am Susan Williams, your nurse practitioner."
Encouragement	Use an open-ended opening statement: "Is there anything you'd like to discuss?" Acknowledge comments: "Yes," and "I understand." Allow silence and observe non-verbal behavior rather than trying to force conversation. Ask for clarification if statements are unclear. Reflect statements back (use sparingly): Patient: "I hate this hospital." Nurse: "You hate this hospital?"
Empathy	Make observations: "You are shaking," and "You seem worried." Recognize feelings: Patient: "I want to go home." Nurse: "It must be hard to be away from your home and family." Provide information as honestly and completely as possible about condition, treatment, and procedures and respond to patient's questions and concerns.

Methods to promote a caring and supportive environment with therapeutic communication include:

Exploration	Verbally express implied messages: Patient: "This treatment is too much trouble." Nurse practitioner: "You think the treatment isn't helping you?" Explore a topic but allow the patient to terminate the discussion without further probing: "I'd like to hear how you feel about that."
Orientation	Indicate reality: Patient: "Someone is screaming." Nurse practitioner: "That sound was an ambulance siren." Comment on distortions without directly agreeing or disagreeing: Patient: "That nurse promised I didn't have to walk again." Nurse: "Really? That's surprising because the doctor ordered physical therapy twice a day."
Collaboration	Work together to achieve better results: "Maybe if we talk about this, we can figure out a way to make the treatment easier for you."
Validation	Seek validation: "Do you feel better now?" or "Did the medication help you breathe better?"

While using therapeutic communication is important, it is equally important to avoid interjecting non-therapeutic communication, which can effectively block effective communication. Avoid the following:

Making negative judgments	"You should stop arguing with the nurses."
Devaluing patient's feelings	"Everyone gets upset at times."
Disagreeing directly	"That can't be true" or "I think you are wrong."
Defending against criticism	"The doctor was not being rude; he's just very busy today."
Changing the subject	This avoids dealing with uncomfortable subjects: Patient: "I'm never going to get well." Nurse: "Your family will be here in a few minutes."
Making inappropriate literal responses	Even as a joke, this is not appropriate, especially if the patient is confused or having difficulty expressing ideas: Patient: "There are bugs crawling under my skin." Nurse: "I'll get some bug spray."
Challenging to establish reality	This often increases confusion and frustration: Patient: "I'm dying!" Nurse: If you were dying, you wouldn't be able to yell and kick."
Stating meaningless clichés	"Don't worry. Everything will be fine." "Isn't it a nice day?"
Providing advice	"You should…" or "The best thing to do is…." It's better when patients ask for advice to provide facts and encourage patients to make their own decisions.
Providing inappropriate approval	This can prevent the patient from expressing true feelings or concerns. Patient: "I shouldn't cry about this." Nurse: "That's right. You're an adult."
Asking for explanations of behavior not directly related to patient care	Asking for explanations such as "Why are you upset?" may require analysis and explanation of feelings on the patient's part.
Agreeing rather than accepting and responding	Agreeing with patient's statements "I agree with you" or "You are right" can make it difficult for the patient to change his/her statement or opinion later.

Nonverbal communication

Non-verbal communication can convey as much information as verbal communication, both on the nurse practitioner's part and the patient's. Non-verbal communication is used for a number of purposes, such as expressing feelings and attitudes, and may be a barrier to communication or a facilitator. While there are cultural differences, interpretation of non-verbal communication can help the nurse to better understand and promote communication:

- Eye contact: Making eye contact provides a connection and shows caring and involvement in the communication. Avoiding contact may indicate someone is not telling the truth or is uncomfortable, fearful, ashamed, or hiding something.
- Tone: The manner in which words are spoken (patiently, cheerfully, somberly) affects the listener, and when the message and tone do not match, it can interfere with communication. A high-pitched tone of voice may indicate nervousness or stress.

- Touch: Reaching out to touch an older adult's hand or pat a shoulder during communication is reassuring but hugging or excessive touching can make people feel uncomfortable. People may touch themselves (lick lips, pick at skin, scratch) if they are anxious.
- Gestures: Using the hands to emphasize meaning is common and may be particularly helpful during explanations, but excessive gesturing can be distracting. Some gestures alone convey message, such as a wave goodbye or pointing. Tapping of the foot, moving the legs, or fidgeting may indicate nervousness. Rubbing the hands together is sometimes a self-comforting measure. Some gestures, such as handshakes, are part of social ritual. Mixed messages, such as fidgeting but speaking with a calm voice, may indicate uncertainty or anxiety.
- Posture: Slumping can indicate lack of interest or withdrawal. Leaning toward the opposite person while talking indicates interest and facilitates interaction.

There are a number of issues related to cultural and spiritual competence in communicating with patients/family:
- Eye contact: Many cultures use eye contact differently than is common in the United States. They may avoid direct eye contact, considering it rude, or may look away to signal disapproval, or may look down to signal respect. Careful observation of the way family members use eye contact can help to determine what will be most comfortable for the patient/family.
- Distance: Some cultures stand close to others (<4 feet) when speaking (Middle Easterners, Hispanics) and others stand at a further distance (>4 feet) (Northern Europeans, many Americans). There is considerable difference relating to concepts of personal space among cultures. Allowing the family to approach or observing whether they tend to move closer, lean forward, or move back can help to determine a comfortable distance for communication.
- Time: Americans tend to be time-oriented, and expect people to be on time, but time is more flexible in many cultures, so scheduling may require flexibility.

Language barriers to communication

Language barriers often compromise patient's access to care and compliance with treatment, especially if the family members are non-English speaking or have poor English skills. If the nurse practitioner's practice draws from a minority population, then the nurse should consider proactive steps to resolving the issue of language barriers, such as hiring bilingual staff, taking language classes, providing translated materials (ie, treatment guidelines and pamphlets), or symbol-based signs. Many practices depend on family members, often children, to translate, but this is not a good solution as children often lack the maturity to assume this responsibility and may also lack the vocabulary or understanding to translate effectively, leading to serious misunderstandings. Interpreters should have training in medical vocabulary. In some cases, volunteer translators can be trained. Another solution is to pool translation resources among a number of practices so that costs are manageable.

Cultural competency

<u>Mexican patients</u>
Many areas of the country have large populations of Mexican and Mexican-Americans. As always, it is important to recognize that cultural generalizations do not always apply to individuals. Recent immigrants, especially, have cultural needs that the nurse practitioner must understand:
- Most Mexicans identify themselves as Catholic and may like the nurse to make arrangements for a priest to visit.
- Large extended families may come to visit to support the patient and family, so patients should receive clear explanations about how many visitors are allowed, but some flexibility may be required.
- Language barriers may exist as some may have limited or no English skills, so translation services should be available around the clock.
- Mexican culture encourages outward expressions of emotions so family may react strongly to news about a patient's condition. Also people who are ill may expect some degree of pampering so extra attention to the patient/family members may alleviate some of their anxiety.

Caring for Mexican patients requires understanding of cultural differences:
- Some immigrant Mexicans have very little formal education, so medical information may seem very complex and confusing, and they may not understand the implications or need for follow-up care.
- Mexican culture perceives time with more flexibility than American culture, so if patients or their family need to be present at a particular time, the nurse practitioner should specify the exact time (1:30 PM) and explain the reason rather than saying something more vague, such as "after lunch."
- People may appear to be unassertive or unable to make decisions when they are simply showing respect to the nurse by being deferent.
- In traditional families, the males make decisions, so women may wait for the husband or other males in the family to make decisions about treatment or care.
- Families may choose to use folk medicine instead of Western medical care or may combine the 2.
- Children and young women are often sheltered and are taught to be respectful to adults, so they may not express their needs openly.

<u>Middle Eastern patients</u>
There are considerable cultural differences among Middle Easterners, but religious beliefs about the segregation of males and females are common. It is important to remember that segregating the female is meant to protect her virtue. Female nurses and nurse practitioners have low status in many countries because they violate this segregation by touching male bodies, so families may not trust or show respect for the female who is caring for their family member. Additionally, male patients may not want to be cared for by female nurses, nurse practitioners, or doctors, and families may be very upset at a female being cared for by a male nurse or physician. When possible, these cultural traditions should be accommodated:
- In Middle Eastern countries, males make decisions, so issues for discussion or decision should be directed to males, such as the spouse or son, and males may be direct in stating what they want, sometimes appearing demanding.

- If a male nurse practitioner must care for a female patient, then the family should be advised that *personal care* (such as bathing) will be done by a female while the medical treatments will be done by the male nurse practitioner.

Caring for Middle Eastern patients requires understanding of cultural differences:
- Families may practice strict dietary restrictions, such as avoiding pork and requiring that animals be killed in a ritual manner, so vegetarian or kosher meals may be required.
- People may have language difficulties often requiring a translator, and same-sex translators should be used if at all possible.
- Patients may be accompanied by large extended families that want to be kept informed and with whom patients consult before decisions are made.
- Most medical care is provided by female relatives, so educating the family about patient care should be directed at females (with female translators if necessary).
- Outward expressions of grief are considered as showing respect for the dead.
- Middle Eastern families often offer gifts to caregivers. Small gifts (candy) should be accepted graciously, but for other gifts, the families should be advised graciously that accepting gifts is against hospital policy.
- Middle Easterners often require less personal space and may stand very close.

Asian patients
There are considerable differences among different Asian populations, so cultural generalizations may not apply to all, but practitioners caring for Asian patients should be aware of common cultural attitudes and behaviors:
- Nurses, nurse practitioners, and doctors are usually viewed with respect, so traditional Asian families may expect the nurse practitioner to remain authoritative and to give directions. Traditional Asian families also may not ask questions, so the nurse should ensure that they understand by having them review material or give demonstrations and should provide explanations clearly, anticipating questions that the family might have but may not articulate.
- Disagreeing is considered impolite. "Yes" may only mean that the person is heard, not that they agree with the person. When asked if they understand, they may indicate that they do even when they clearly do not, so as not to offend the practitioner.
- Asians may avoid eye contact as an indication of respect.

Caring for Asian patients requires understanding of cultural differences:
- Patients/families may not show outward expressions of feelings/grief, sometimes appearing passive. They also avoid public displays of affection. This does not mean that they don't feel, just that they don't show their feelings.
- Families often hide illness and disabilities from others and may feel ashamed about illness.
- Terminal illness is often hidden from the patient, so family may not want patients to know they are dying or seriously ill.
- Families may use cupping, pinching, or applying pressure to injured areas, and this can leave bruises that may appear as abuse, so when bruises are found, the family should be questioned about alternative therapy before assumptions are made.
- Patients may be treated with traditional herbs.
- Families may need translators because of poor or no English skills.
- In traditional Asian families, males are authoritative and make the decisions.

Gay, lesbian, bisexual, and transgendered patients

Gay, lesbian, bisexual, and transgendered patients often experience hostility and discrimination because of their sexual identification. Some experience anxiety and stress when coming to terms with their sexuality and/or when coming out to family or friends. Increasingly, adolescents are self-identifying as homosexual, some as early as age 12, and they may face intense pressure from family and peers. Homosexual/transgendered military personnel must deal with the fear of being identified and losing their careers. Hate crimes against homosexual/transgendered people continue. Children of gay/lesbian parents may face discrimination as well. While some religious groups and therapists recommend "reparation" therapy to convert homosexuals to heterosexuals, the American Psychiatric Association (APA) opposes such therapy, and evidence suggests it is virtually never successful and can be damaging psychologically. The nurse practitioner must respect the individual's sexual identification, remain supportive, and should be knowledgeable about issues important to gay, lesbian, bisexual, and transgendered patients. The rights and needs of partners should also be respected.

Collaboration with patient and families

One of the most important forms of collaboration is that between the nurse practitioner and the patient/family, but this type of collaboration is often overlooked. Nurse practitioners and others in the healthcare team must always remember that the point of collaborating is to improve patient care, and this means that the patient and patient's family must remain central to all planning. For example, including family in planning for a patient takes time initially, but sitting down and asking the patient and family, "What do you want?" and using the synergy model to evaluate patient's (and family's) characteristics can provide valuable information that saves time in the long run and facilitates planning and expenditure of resources. Families, and even young children, often want to participate in care and planning and feel validated and more positive toward the medical system when they are included.

Self-awareness

The nurse practitioner must develop a self-awareness of personal values, biases, motivating forces, beliefs, strengths, weaknesses, feelings, and attitudes because these all color interactions with patients. If, for example, a patient senses prejudice, the patient may react negatively to this. In some cases, the nurse practitioner's personal beliefs about others may affect a patient evaluation when the nurse makes judgments based on personal feelings rather than clinical observations. A strong self-awareness based on honest exploration can be an asset when working with the patient as it can guide the nurse practitioner's behavior and responses to better promote a therapeutic relationship. The nurse must be able to maintain a personal sense of values while respecting those with different value systems. Nurse practitioners can increase self-awareness by maintaining a journal of feelings, discussing values with others and seeking to understand those with differing values and beliefs, and working with a mentor.

Therapeutic relationship

A therapeutic relationship is a continuum based on a trusting relationship, caring, empathy, and acceptance. The needs of the patient are the focus, not the feelings or needs of the nurse practitioner:
- Orientation: The patient seeks or is brought in for help, and needs and concerns are elicited.

- Nurse practitioner responds to client, listens actively, and responds, explaining roles and trying to relieve the patient's anxiety while helping the patient focus on problems.
- Identification: The patient begins to identify with the nurse practitioner and increases understanding of problems and testing behavior decreases as the patient has a better understanding of roles and expectations.
- The nurse shows acceptance and continues to assess and provide support and information.
- Working: The patient makes better use of the relationship, shows better problem-solving skills, and improved communication, but may engage in exploitative behavior (with wide behavior shifts in dependence and independence).
- Nurse supports client and explores feelings at client's own pace.
- Termination: The patient establishes independence from nurse and sets new goals.

The nurse encourages family/community support and preventive care.

Building and maintaining a trusting relationship

It is essential that the nurse practitioner builds and maintains a trusting relationship with the patient by respecting the individual and maintaining confidentiality. Patients are often stressed and frightened and may express this through criticizing, withdrawing, or refusing to cooperate; the nurse practitioner should not react negatively but should remain supportive and encourage communication. The nurse should take the time to understand the cultural needs of the patient and to ensure that the nurse's own personal preferences don't interfere with provision of care. The patient's healthcare issues should be viewed from the patient's perspective. If the nurse practitioner must rush out of the patient's room, the practitioner should explain why he/she is rushed and return at a later time. Using the patient's name routinely and taking even a minute or two to talk to the patient can help to reassure the patient and build trust.

Nurse practitioner-patient relationship

The nurse practitioner-patient relationship is a delicate marriage of skill, ethics, and trust. It is a particularly vulnerable relationship in a psychotherapy setting, as the nurse and patient discuss a wide range of negative experiences, thoughts, and family history. Nurse and patient must respect each other, even though they may not like one another. The nurse practitioner motivates and empowers the patient towards lifestyle change and therapeutic compliance. In a mental health setting, the nurse practitioner is responsible for the overall health and well being of the patient, so conditions must be established under which rules are enforced and privileges are awarded. The nurse practitioner is legally responsible for reporting to the police when he/she fears for the patient's life or that of another individual. The practitioner must not allow personal feelings for the patient to affect his/her treatment or professional recommendations and, if unable to deal with personal emotions, should inform a colleague and refer the patient to another competent individual.

Therapeutic alliance

The therapeutic alliance between the patient and the nurse practitioner is a critical aspect of a therapeutic relationship. This alliance involves:
- Goals: Collaboration in treatment goals is essential because it forms a partnership between the nurse practitioner and the patient.

- Tasks: Both the nurse practitioner and the patient should have an understanding of the tasks required of them.
- Bond: Over time, a personal relationship and bond develops as patient and nurse work to achieve goals.

The strength of the therapeutic alliance directly relates to the treatment outcomes. Factors that affect the alliance include qualities of the nurse, qualities of the patient, and aspects of therapy. Patients who have demonstrated difficulty establishing relationships in their personal lives sometimes also have difficulty establishing a therapeutic alliance with a mental healthcare provider. Showing respect for the patient, showing sensitivity to culture, and asking the patient for input can strengthen the alliance.

Termination

The final stage of the patient-provider relationship is the termination or resolution phase. The nurse should establish the basis for termination of treatment at the onset. Reasons for termination may include non-compliance with treatment, reaching therapeutic goals, or referral and should be explained verbally and in writing. Termination can be very difficult for both the patient and the provider. The patient must now focus on continuing without the guiding assistance of the therapy. The patient will need to utilize newfound approaches and behaviors. This time may be one of varying emotions for the patient who may be reluctant to end the relationship. The patient may experience anxiety, anger, or sadness. The provider may need to guide the patient in utilizing newfound strategies in dealing with feelings about the termination of the relationship. Focus should be placed on the future.

Literacy assessment

A literacy assessment should be part of the initial interview with the patient. Basic information can be gleaned by having the patient fill out a simple form about history and educational background, if possible, as this demonstrates the patient's ability to read basic questions and provides literacy information. The nurse practitioner should pay close attention to the patient's vocabulary and syntax as this correlates with literacy, although those with learning disabilities may be able to express themselves well but still have difficulty reading. The nurse must use language that the patient understands, so assessing health literacy is equally important. The nurse can begin by asking patients what they know about their illnesses. Even with well-educated patients, the nurse practitioner should use common terms rather than medical terms whenever possible as patients may not tell the nurse if they don't understand.

Patient education on safely taking prescription medications

Patient education is vital to the success and safety of taking prescription medications. Patient education should include both the generic and brand name of the drug, indications for use, expected actions of the drug, dosage, route and duration of effects, what to do when a dose is missed, any associated precautions (i.e., operating machinery or diet restrictions), any associated side effects, and when to call the prescribing medical practitioner or seek help. Patients should also be educated on ways to help decrease side effects. They should be given written information including drug name, dosage, action, side effects, purpose, and any other pertinent information about the specific medication. All patient education should be documented, including a patient's understanding of the information, evaluation of patient's ability to administer the medication, and ability to obtain the medication.

Professional Role and Policy

Leadership styles

Leadership styles often influence the perception of leadership values and commitment to collaboration. There are a number of different leadership styles:

Charismatic	Depends upon personal charisma to influence people, and may be very persuasive, but this type leader may engage "followers" and relate to one group rather than the organization at large, limiting effectiveness.
Bureaucratic	Follows organization rules exactly and expects everyone else to do so. This is most effective in handling cash flow or managing work in dangerous work environments. This type of leadership may engender respect but may not be conducive to change.
Autocratic	Makes decisions independently and strictly enforces rules, but team members often feel left out of process and may not be supportive. This type of leadership is most effective in crisis situations, but may have difficulty gaining commitment of staff
Consultative	Presents a decision and welcomes input and questions although decisions rarely change. This type of leadership is most effective when gaining the support of staff is critical to the success of proposed changes.
Participatory	Presents a potential decision and then makes final decision based on input from staff or teams. This type of leadership is time-consuming and may result in compromises that are not wholly satisfactory to management or staff, but this process is motivating to staff who feel their expertise is valued.
Democratic	Presents a problem and asks staff or teams to arrive at a solution although the leader usually makes the final decision. This type of leadership may delay decision-making, but staff and teams are often more committed to the solutions because of their input.
Laissez-faire (free rein)	Exerts little direct control but allows employees/ teams to make decisions with little interference. This may be effective leadership if teams are highly skilled and motivated, but in many cases this type of leadership is the product of poor management skills and little is accomplished because of this lack of leadership.

Networking

Networking is the act of meeting others in order to make mutually beneficial connections. The nurse practitioner should attend local, state, and national conferences. Conferences offer the opportunity to network, build skills, and refresh an organization's style. An essential aspect of business is networking. Effective networking involves speaking with others and learning about their services and ideas. Sharing contact information is a must when networking. Conferences also offer nurse practitioners the opportunity to learn new skills and approaches to various situations, and to comply with national standards. Conferences offer nurse practitioners opportunities for personal professional development, so that he/she will be more knowledgeable. Conferences also allow the nurse an opportunity to gain recognition for his/her research and/or the institution he/she represents.

Communication skills needed for leading intra- and interdisciplinary teams

A number of communication skills are needed to lead and facilitate coordination of intra- and interdisciplinary teams, such as the following:

- Communicating openly is essential with all members encouraged to participate as valued members of a cooperative team.
- Avoiding interrupting or interpreting the point another is trying to make allows free flow of ideas.
- Avoiding jumping to conclusions as this can effectively shut off communication.
- Active listening requires paying attention and asking questions for clarification rather than challenging the ideas of others.
- Respecting the opinions and ideas of others, even when they are opposed to one's own, is absolutely essential.
- Reacting and responding to facts rather than feelings allows one to avoid angry confrontations or diffuse anger.
- Clarifying information or opinions stated can help avoid misunderstandings.
- Keeping unsolicited advice out of the conversation shows respect for others and allows them to solicit advice without feeling pressured.

Promoting collaboration

Promoting collaboration and assisting others to understand and use resources and expertise of others requires a commitment in terms of time and effort. Examples of promoting collaboration include:

- Coaching others on methods of collaboration can include providing information in the form of handouts about effective communication strategies and, in turn, modeling this type of communication with the staff being coached.
- Team meetings are commonly held on nursing units and provide an opportunity to model collaboration and suggest the need for outside expertise to help with planning patient care plans. The mentoring nurse practitioner can initiate discussions about resources that are available in the facility or the community.
- Selecting a diverse group for teams or inviting those with expertise in various areas to join the team when needed can help team members to appreciate and understand how to use the input of other resources.

Interdisciplinary collaboration

Interdisciplinary collaboration is absolutely critical to practice if the needs and best interests of the patients and families are central. Interdisciplinary practice begins with nurse practitioners and physicians but extends to pharmacists, social workers, occupational and physical therapists, nutritionists, and a wide range of allied healthcare providers, all of whom cooperate in diagnosis and treatment; however, state regulations determine to some degree how much autonomy a nurse practitioner can have in diagnosing and treating. While nurses have increasingly gained more legal rights, they have also become more dependent upon collaboration with others for their expertise and for referrals if the patient's needs extend beyond the nurse practitioner's ability to provide assistance. Additionally, the prescriptive ability of nurse practitioners varies from state to state, with some requiring direct supervision by other disciplines (such as physicians), while others require particular types of supervisory arrangements, depending upon the circumstances.

Intra- and interdisciplinary teams

The complexity of patient care requires collaboration among intra- and interdisciplinary teams. Collaboration may begin between the nurse practitioner and patient, but often the expertise of others in the healthcare community must be included. Often the nurse practitioner is in the position to seek collaboration and to recognize when multiple perspectives can be helpful in solving conflicts or making decisions about health care. Collaboration requires open sharing of ideas and respect for the expertise of the individual. Collaboration requires more than just talking, however. In many cases it may be more formalized, with specialized committees formed in order to solve specific problems. Studies have indicated that patients benefit from collaborative efforts between nurse and physician, and this benefit extends to others as well. In a collaborative environment, all of the participants benefit from sharing ideas and discussion that can lead to innovative problem solving.

Synergy model of collaboration

The Synergy model of collaboration is a team approach of working with a variety of others (physicians, nurses, dieticians, therapist, families, social workers, community leaders and members, clergy, intra- and interdisciplinary teams) in a cooperative manner, using good therapeutic communication skills, to ensure that each person is contributing optimally toward reaching patient goals and positive outcomes. Collaboration requires mutual respect, professional maturity, common purpose, and a positive sense of self. Levels of collaboration include:

- Level 1: This nurse participates in collaborative activities, learns from others (including mentors), and respects the input of others.
- Level 3: This nurse not only participates in collaborative activities but also initiates them and actively seeks learning opportunities.
- Level 5: This nurse takes a leadership role in collaborative activities by mentoring and teaching others while still seeking learning opportunities and actively seeks additional resources as needed.

Contract for services

A nurse practitioner working as an independent contractor may sign a contract for services, a legal financial agreement that outlines the conditions of service. Typically, a contract includes:

- The name of the nurse practitioner and the client, outlining the qualifications, appropriate licensure, and/or certification.
- Purpose of the service agreement.
- Contract period, including beginning date and ending date of the contract.
- Compensation, including daily, weekly, or hourly rate of payment.
- Expenses, such as travel pay or money for office support, equipment, or training and methods of submitting invoices.
- Performance description outlining the type of services that the independent contractor will perform, including any limitations and legal responsibilities.
- Disclaimers.

Consultant

The mental health professional often serves as a consultant to others, especially during discharge planning, to ensure that patients receive the continued care and services that they need. The nurse practitioner may serve as an educational consultant, providing general information about the needs of those with psychiatric or mental health issues, or may specifically deal with the needs of a particular patient, in which case the nurse must be sure that proper release forms have been signed and issues of privacy are respected. Areas of consultation include:

- Schools: The school nurse or educators may require information on dealing with behavioral or treatment issues.
- Housing: If a patient is placed in housing such as board-and-care homes or supervised apartments, authorities need to understand the patient's condition and needs.
- Social Services: The nurse may provide consultation services to social workers. If a child is placed in foster care, the foster parents should be provided information necessary to provide care and support to the child.

Collaboration with external agencies

The nurse practitioner must initiate and facilitate collaboration with external agencies because many have direct impacts on patient care and needs:

- Industry can include other facilities sharing interests in patient care or pharmaceutical companies. It's important for nursing to have a dialog with drug companies about their products and how they are used in specific populations because many medications are prescribed to women, children, or the aged without validating studies for dose or efficacy.
- Payors have a vested interest in containing health care costs, so providing information and representing the interests of the patient is important.
- Community groups may provide resources for patients and families, both in terms of information and financial or other assistance.
- Political agencies are increasingly important as new laws are considered about nurse-patient ratios and infection control in many states.
- Public health agencies are partners in health care with other facilities and must be included, especially in issues related to communicable disease.

Resistance to organizational change

Performance improvement processes cannot occur without organizational change, and resistance to change is common for many people, so coordinating collaborative processes requires anticipating resistance and taking steps to achieve cooperation. Resistance often relates to concerns about job loss, increased responsibilities, and general denial or lack of understanding and frustration.

Leaders can prepare others involved in the process of change by taking these steps:

- Be honest, informative, and tactful, giving people thorough information about anticipated changes and how the changes will affect them, including positives.
- Be patient in allowing people the time they need to contemplate changes and express anger or disagreement.
- Be empathetic in listening carefully to the concerns of others.
- Encourage participation, allowing staff to propose methods of implementing change, so they feel some sense of ownership.

- Establish a climate in which all staff members are encouraged to identify the need for change on an ongoing basis.
- Present further ideas for change to management.

Conflict resolution

Conflict is an almost inevitable product of collaboration with the patient, and the nurse practitioner must assume responsibility for conflict resolution. While conflicts can be disruptive, they can produce positive outcomes by forcing people to listen to different perspectives and opening dialogue. The nurse practitioner should make a plan for dealing with conflict resolution. The best time for conflict resolution is when differences emerge but before open conflict and hardening of positions occur. The nurse practitioner must pay close attention to the people and problems involved, listen carefully, and reassure those involved that their points of view are understood. Steps to conflict resolution include:
- Allow both sides to present their side of conflict without bias, maintaining a focus on opinions rather than individuals.
- Encourage cooperation through negotiation and compromise.
- Maintain the focus, providing guidance to keep the discussions on track, and avoid arguments.
- Evaluate the need for renegotiation, formal resolution process, or third party.
- Utilize humor and empathy to diffuse escalating tensions.
- Summarize the issues, outlining key arguments.
- Avoid forcing resolution if possible

Professional boundaries

Professional boundaries that show respect for the individual can be difficult to establish as part of delivery of care, especially with diverse populations because the nurse practitioner may unknowingly violate personal or spiritual values. Diverse groups include those on the fringes of society, such as the homeless or the abused. It's very important that nurse practitioners remain cognizant of the potential to abuse a position of power in which the patient and family are in many ways dependent upon the nurse practitioner and because of language, fears, or cultural constraints may not feel able to state their concerns. A relationship with a patient must be caring but at the same time professional and non-judgmental. The needs of the patient/family must always be considered, and this may mean utilizing a translator to ensure that the patient/family are assuming an active role in the plan of care or making referrals to others in the healthcare or allied professions.

Patients' rights

Patients' (families') rights in relation to what they should expect from a healthcare organization are outlined in both standards of the Joint Commission and National Committee for Quality Assurance. Rights include:
- Respect for patient, including personal dignity and psychosocial, spiritual, and cultural considerations.
- Response to needs related to access and pain control.
- Ability to make decisions about care, including informed consent, advance directives, and end-of-life care.
- Procedure for registering complaints or grievances.

- Protection of confidentiality and privacy.
- Freedom from abuse or neglect.
- Protection during research and information related to ethical issues of research.
- Appraisal of outcomes, including unexpected outcomes.
- Information about organization, services, and practitioners.
- Appeal procedures for decisions regarding benefits and quality of care.
- Organizational code of ethical behavior.
- Procedures for donating and procuring organs/tissue.

Negligence

Risk management must attempt to determine the burden of proof for acts of negligence, including compliance with duty, breaches in procedures, degree of harm, and cause. Negligence indicates that proper care has not been provided, based on established standards. Reasonable care uses rationale for decision-making in relation to providing care. State regulations regarding negligence may vary but all have some statutes of limitation. There are a number of different types of negligence:
- Negligent conduct indicates that an individual failed to provide reasonable care or to protect/assist another, based on standards and expertise.
- Gross negligence is willfully providing inadequate care while disregarding the safety and security of another.
- Contributory negligence involves the injured party contributing to his/her own harm.
- Comparative negligence attempts to determine what percentage amount of negligence is attributed to each individual involved.

CQI

Continuous Quality Improvement (CQI) emphasizes the organization and systems and processes within that organization rather than individuals. It recognizes internal customers (staff) and external customers (patients) and utilizes data to improve processes. CQI represents the concept that most processes can be improved. CQI uses the scientific method of experimentation to meet needs and improve services and utilizes various tools, such as brainstorming, multivoting, various charts and diagrams, storyboarding, and meetings.

Core concepts include:
- Quality and success, defined as meeting or exceeding internal and external customer's needs and expectations.
- Problems relate to processes, and variations in process lead to variations in results.
- Change can be in small steps.

Steps to CQI include:
- Forming a knowledgeable team.
- Identifying and defining measures used to determine success.
- Brainstorming strategies for change.
- Plan, collect, and utilize data as part of making decisions.
- Test changes and revise or refine as needed.

QI

Quality improvement (QI) is accomplished through peer review or another form of assessment. In peer review, the approach is to acknowledge and prize the work nurses do. This shows the way toward better standards of work and puts off work that is not within what the practitioner can legally do. It heightens the quality of medical attention and gives a means for attaining answerability and conscientiousness. Another form of assessment may include an audit, question/answer or appraisal, or patient contentment question/answer or appraisal.

Risk management – Organizations and actions meant to acknowledge and intercede resulting in less chance of harm to a patient and ensuing claims in opposition to the medical attention workers. This is founded on the supposition that a lot of harm done to patients could be stopped from happening in the first place. Risk management is an assessment of places when legal responsibility is an issue, like patients, methods, or how accounts are maintained. Risk management also involves instruction used to lessen the chance of a problem in a recognized part.

Integration of key quality concepts within the organization

There are a number of key concepts related to quality that must be communicated to all members of an organization through inservice, workshops, newsletters, fact sheets, and team meetings. Quality care/performance should be:
- Appropriate to needs and in keeping with best practices.
- Accessible to the individual despite financial, cultural, or other barriers.
- Competent, with practitioners well-trained and adhering to standards.
- Coordinated among all healthcare providers.
- Effective in achieving outcomes based on the current state of knowledge.
- Efficient in methods of achieving the desired outcomes.
- Preventive, allowing for early detection and prevention of problems.
- Respectful and caring with consideration of the individual needs given primary importance.
- Safe so that the organization is free of hazards or dangers that may put patients or others at risk.

Factors necessary for information quality

Quality information is defined by the following factors:
- Timeliness: The necessary data is available (and retrievable) as needed.
- Precision: System dictionaries shall describe uniform wording and clear definitions.
- Accuracy: The data should be as error-free as possible.
- Measurability: The information should be quantifiable so that comparisons can be made.
- Independently verifiable: The integrity of the information remains constant regardless of the individual reporting it.
- Availability: The information should be accessible where it is needed. In the hospital or clinic environment, the information should usually be available at the patient's location.

Integrating the results of data analysis

Integrating the results of data analysis is necessary because attempting performance improvement and developing practice guidelines without data is essentially operating blind. This data should be used not only as the basis for long-term strategic planning but for identifying opportunities for performance improvement activities on an ongoing basis. Integration of information includes:
- Identifying issues for tracking.
- Reviewing patterns and trends to determine how they impact care.
- Establishing action plans and desired outcomes based on the need for improvement.
- Providing information to process improvement teams to facilitate change.
- Evaluating systems and processes for follow-up.
- Monitoring specific cases, criteria, critical pathways, and outcomes.

The integration of information should assist with case management, decision making about patient care, improvement of critical pathways related to clinical performance, staff performance evaluations, as well as credentialing and privileging.

Discharge planning

Discharge planning should begin on admission and must be a joint effort so that the transfer and discharge documents provide the information that the individual or staff at transfer facilities/home need. Information should include:
- Contact telephone numbers, e-mail addresses, and street addresses for the nurse practitioner (to contact patient for discharge surveillance) and patient or transfer facility staff (to contact nurse practitioner if problems arise).
- Information sheets outlining signs for all risk factors, especially if patient is discharged to their home without nursing care.
- Follow-up appointment dates, with physicians, labs, or the nurse practitioner.
- Specific directions for medication or treatments, including side effects.
- Information about 12-step/self-help/community-assistance programs.

Patients who are homeless require further assistance with discharge, as compliance with treatment and follow-up appointments is poor in the homeless population. Homeless patients should receive:
- Lists of safe shelters and places they can go to bathe, eat, and get mail.
- Assistance in applying for welfare assistance or Social Security.

Safety and decision-making

In 2005, Ebright et al published a study of factors related to safety and the decision-making ability of the nurse practitioner. Every clinical decision made by the nurse practitioner has an effect on the safety of the patient, and therefore any factor that influences the nurse practitioner's decision-making ability may adversely affect the patient. Ebright at al identified the following factors that influence decision-making and patient safety: knowledge base, attention, barriers to care, number of tasks, missing essential information, and behaviors that are not encouraging of productive thought. The presence of, or a change in, any of these factors can result in unnecessary harm for the patient.

Evidence-based best-practice guidelines

Evidence-based best-practice guidelines apply the use of best practices for such things as standing medicine orders or antibiotic protocols that are in common use, but decisions are often made based on studies that lack internal and/or external validity or on expert opinion colored by personal bias, so the process of establishing evidence-based best-practice guidelines should be done systematically. Including those who are resistive to the process often helps to facilitate the establishment of guidelines, but it is important that decisions be made on solid evidence as much as possible. Simply dispensing evidence-based best-practice guidelines often does not change practice, so consideration must be given to implementation. Decisions must be made as to whether the use of the guidelines is mandatory (standing orders) and to what degree individual practitioners can choose other options. Guidelines that are too rigid may be counter-productive. In some case, establishing guidelines may affect cost-reimbursement from third-party payers.

Steps to developing evidence-based best-practice guidelines include:
- Focus on the topic/methodology: This includes outlining possible interventions/treatments for review, choosing patient populations and settings, and determining significant outcomes. Search boundaries (such as types of journals, types of studies, dates of studies) should be determined.
- Evidence review: This includes review of literature, critical analysis of studies, and summarizing of results, including pooled meta-analysis.
- Expert judgment: Recommendations based on personal experience from a number of experts may be utilized, especially if there is inadequate evidence based on review, but this subjective evidence should be explicitly acknowledged.
- Policy considerations: This includes cost-effectiveness, access to care, insurance coverage, availability of qualified staff, and legal implications.
- Policy: A written policy must be completed with recommendations. Common practice is to utilize letter guidelines, with "A" the most highly recommended, usually based on the quality of supporting evidence.
- Review: The completed policy should be submitted to peers for review and comments before instituting the policy.

Critical analysis

The nurse practitioner must be taught and understand the process of critical analysis and know how to conduct a survey of the literature. Basic concepts related to research include:
- Survey of valid sources: Information from a juried journal and an anonymous or personal website are very different sources, and evaluating what constitutes a valid source of data is critical.
- Evaluation of internal and external validity: Internal validity shows a cause and effect relationship between 2 variables, with the cause occurring before the effect and no intervening variable. External validity occurs when results hold true in different environments and circumstances with different populations.
- Sample selection and sample size: Selection and size can have a huge impact on the results, but a sample that is too small may lack both internal and external validity. Selection may be so narrowly focused that the results can't be generalized to other groups.

Identifying clinical problems amenable to research

Identifying clinical problems amenable to research is an evolving skill. Inexperienced nurse practitioners, especially those just starting out in nursing practice, are often looking to build information and skills because they lack experiential learning. They may research information about a disease or treatment that they are dealing with in order to have better skills and understanding. More experienced nurse practitioners, on the other hand, often look for information to improve patient outcomes, such as researching new procedures, treatments, or equipment for broader application. However, there is a need for both. Clinical inquiry is a program of questioning and evaluating practice through research and experience. It should include seeking a variety of data on a topic, evaluating the data, pooling results, and making determinations as to validity or applicability to the clinical practice. Clinical inquiry is also part of evidence-based practice in which data is used to support clinical decisions on an ongoing basis.

Internal and external validity, generalizability, and replication

Many research studies are most concerned with internal validity, adequate unbiased data properly collected and analyzed within the population studied, but studies that determine the efficacy of procedures or treatments, for example, should have external validity as well; that is, the results should be generalizable (true) for similar populations. Replication of the study with different subjects, researchers, and under different circumstances should produce similar results. For various reasons, some people may be excluded from a study so that instead of randomized subjects the subjects may be highly selected, so when data is compared with another population, in which there is less or more selection, results may be different. The selection of subjects, in this case, would interfere with external validity. Part of the design of a study should include considerations of whether or not it should have external validity or whether there is value for the institution based solely on internal validation.

Selection and information bias

Selection bias occurs when the method of selecting subjects results in a cohort that is not representative of the target population because of inherent error in design. For example, if all patients who develop urinary infections are evaluated per urine culture and sensitivities for microbial resistance, but only those patients with clinically-evident infections are included, a number of patients with sub-clinical infections may be missed, skewing the results. Selection bias is only a concern when participants in studies are specifically chosen. Many surveillance studies do not involve selection of subjects. Information bias occurs when there are errors in classification, so an estimate of association is incorrect. Non-differential misclassification occurs when there is similar misclassification of disease or exposure among both those who are diseased/exposed and those who are not. Differential misclassification occurs when there is a differing misclassification of disease or exposure among both those who are diseased/exposed and those who are not.

Population and sampling

Defining the population is critical to data collection and the criteria must be established early in the process. The population may comprise a particular group of individuals, objects, or events. In some cases, data is gathered on an entire population, such as all cases with a particular disease, all deaths, or all physicians in a particular discipline, usually within a specified time frame. In other cases, sampling, using a subset of a population, may be done to measure only part of a given population and to generalize the findings to the larger target population while accurately representing the target population. There are a number of considerations with sampling:

- The sampling must have the characteristics of the target population.
- The design of the collection must specify the size of the sample, the location, and time period.
- The sampling technique must ensure that the sampling represents the target population accurately.
- The design of the collection must ensure that the sampling will not be biased.

Tracking and trending

Tracking and trending are central to developing research-supported evidence-based practice and is part of continuous quality improvement. Once processes and outcomes measurements are selected, then at least 1 measure should be tracked for a number of periods of time, usually in increments of 4 weeks or quarterly. This tracking can be used to present graphical representation of results that will show trends. While trends will show some normal variation, if the trend becomes erratic and measures are inconsistent, this suggests that the processes of care are not consistent or are inadequate. For example, if infections in peripherally inserted central catheter (PICC) lines are tracked and the trend shows wild fluctuations with high levels of infection in 1 period, low in another, and vacillations in a third, then the first step is to ensure that the process is being followed correctly. If the process is stable but the variations persist, then the next course would be to modify the process by looking at best practices.

Risk stratification

Risk stratification involves statistical adjustment to account for confounding and differences in risk factors. Confounding issues are those that confuse the data outcomes, such as trying to compare different populations, different ages, or different genders. For example, if there are 2 physicians and 1 has primarily high-risk patients, and the other has primarily low-risk patients, the same rate of infection (by raw data) would suggest that the infection risks are equal for both physicians' patients. However, high-risk patients are much more prone to infection, so in this case risk stratification to account for this difference would show that the patients of the physician with low-risk patients had a much higher risk of infection, relatively speaking. Risk stratification is also used to predict outcomes of surgery by accounting for various risk factors (including ASO score, age, and medical conditions). Risk stratification is an important element of data analysis.

Hypothesis and hypothesis testing

A hypothesis should be generated about the probable cause of the disease/infection based on the information available in laboratory and medical records, epidemiologic study, literature review, and expert opinion. A hypothesis, for example, should include the infective agent, the likely source, and the mode of transmission: "Wound infections with *Staphylococcus aureus* were caused by reuse and inadequate sterilization of single-use irrigation syringes used during wound care in the ICU." Hypothesis testing includes data analysis, laboratory findings, and outcomes of environmental testing. It usually includes case control studies, with 2-4 controls picked for each case of infection. They may be matched according to age, sex, or other characteristics, but they are not infected at the time they are picked for the study. Cohort studies, whose controls are picked based on having or lacking exposure, may also be instituted. If the hypothesis cannot be supported, then a new hypothesis or different testing methods may be necessary.

Evidence-based research

Evidence-based research is the use of current research and patient values in practice to establish a plan of care for each patient. Research may be the result of large studies of best practices or individual research from observations in practice about the effectiveness of treatment. Evidence-based practice requires a commitment to ongoing research and outcomes evaluations. Many resources are available:

- Guide to Clinical Preventive Services by the Agency for Healthcare Research and Quality of the U.S. Department of Health and Human Services (http://www.ahrq.gov/clinic/cps3dix.htm).

Evidence-based practice requires a thorough understanding of research methods in order to evaluate the results and determine if they can be generalized. Results must also be evaluated in terms of cost-effectiveness. Steps to evidence-based practice include:

- Making a diagnosis.
- Researching and analyzing results.
- Applying research findings to plan of care.
- Evaluating outcomes.

Data definition and collection of data

Data definitions must be based on a solid understanding of statistical analysis and epidemiological concepts. Specific issues that must be addressed include:

- The 3 Ss:
  - Sensitivity: The data should include all positive cases, taking into account variables, decreasing the number of false negatives.
  - Specificity: The data should include only those cases specific to the needs of the measurement and exclude those that may be similar but are a different population, decreasing the number of false positives.
  - Stratification: Date should be classified according to subsets, taking variables into consideration.
- 2 Rs:
  - Recordability: The tool/indicator should collect and measure the necessary data.
  - Reliability: Results should be reproducible.
- UV:
  - Usability: The tool or indicator should be easy to utilize and understand.
  - Validity: Collection should measure the target adequately, so that the results have predictive value.

Outcomes data

Outcomes data provides an effective guide for performance improvement activities because it gives evidence of how well a process succeeds but not necessarily the reason; therefore, outcomes data must be evaluated accordingly. There are inherent problems with outcome data that must be considered when utilizing outcomes for process improvement. First, it is almost impossible to provide sufficient risk stratification to provide complete validity to outcomes data, and, second, it is also difficult to accurately attribute the outcomes data to any 1 step in a process without further study. For example, if outcomes data show a decline in deaths in the emergency department, which recently changed trauma procedures, but doesn't account for the fact that a gang task force has successfully decreased drive-by shootings and killings by 70%, it might be assumed that changes in the emergency department altered the outcome data when, in fact, if the data were adjusted for these external factors, the death rate may have increased.

When interpreting outcomes data, one should keep in mind that there are a number of different types of outcomes data to be considered, and some data may overlap:
- Clinical: This includes symptoms, diagnoses, staging of disease, and indicators of patient health.
- Physiological: This includes measures of physical abnormalities, loss of function, and activities of daily living.
- Psychosocial: This includes feelings, perceptions, beliefs, functional impairment, and role performance.
- Integrative: This includes measures of mortality, longevity, and cost-effectiveness.
- Perception: This includes customer perceptions, evaluations, and satisfaction.
- Organization-wide clinical: This includes readmissions, adverse reactions, and deaths.

When considering outcomes data, the focus may be on the process or just the outcomes data, and the team analyzing the data should clarify the purpose of reviewing the data and should understand how process and outcomes data interrelate.

Evidence-based practice

Evidence-based practice is the use of current research and individual values in practice to establish a plan of care for each individual. Research may be the result of large studies of best practices or individual research from observations in practice about the effectiveness of treatment. Evidence-based practice requires a commitment to ongoing research and outcomes evaluations. Many resources are available, such as the *Guide to Clinical Preventive Services* by the Agency for Healthcare Research and Quality of the U. S. Department of Health and Human Services (http://www.ahrq.gov/clinic/cps3dix.htm). Evidence-based practice requires a thorough understanding of research methods to evaluate the results and determine if they can be generalized. Results must also be evaluated in terms of cost-effectiveness. Steps to evidence-based practice include:
- Making a diagnosis.
- Researching and analyzing results.
- Applying research findings to a plan of care.
- Evaluating outcomes.

Steps to developing guidelines
Steps to developing evidence-based practice guidelines include the following:
- Focus on the topic/methodology: This includes outlining possible interventions/treatments for review, choosing individual populations and settings, and determining significant outcomes. Search boundaries (e.g., journals, studies, dates of studies) should be determined.
- Evidence review: This includes review of literature, critical analysis of studies, and a summary of results, including pooled meta-analysis.
- Expert judgment: Recommendations based on personal experience from a number of experts may be used, especially if there is inadequate evidence based on review, but this subjective evidence should be explicitly acknowledged.
- Policy considerations: This includes cost-effectiveness, access to care, insurance coverage, availability of qualified staff, and legal implications.

- Policy: A written policy must be completed with recommendations. Common practice is to use letter guidelines, with "A" the most highly recommended, usually based on the quality of supporting evidence.
- Review: The completed policy should be submitted to peers for review and comments before instituting the policy.

Strategies

Evidence-based practice must be part of the mission and goal of a health care organization, and strategies to attain this must be supported at all levels. Information technology tools, such as Internet capability or access to information databases, should be available at the point of care so that health care providers are able to access journal articles and other clinical information. Links may be available through the patient's health risk evaluation as well. All staff should receive training in the use of equipment and methods of researching and retrieving information and have an understanding of how to interpret research findings; the inability of health care providers to understand and interpret findings can be a significant barrier to evidence-based practice. Because evidence-based practice often results in change, institutional support for change must be evident and may involve incentives. Continuing education classes should be available on-site to help health care providers gain the research skills they need.

Outcome evaluation

Outcomes evaluation is an important component of evidence-based practice, which involves both internal and external research. All treatments are subjected to review to determine if they produce positive outcomes, and policies and protocols for outcomes evaluation should be in place. Outcomes evaluation includes the following:
- Monitoring over the course of treatment involves careful observation and record keeping that notes progress, with supporting laboratory and radiographic evidence as indicated by condition and treatment.
- Evaluating results includes reviewing records as well as current research to determine if outcomes are within acceptable parameters.
- Sustaining involves continuing treatment, but continuing to monitor and evaluate.
- Improving means to continue the treatment but with additions or modifications in order to improve outcomes.
- Replacing the treatment with a different treatment must be done if outcomes evaluation indicates that current treatment is ineffective.

Incorporation of research findings

Incorporating research findings should be central to all work of the nurse practitioner and should be routinely disseminated as part of practice, education, and consultation. Any time the nurse gives a presentation or provides written material, references should be made to research findings because this provides supporting evidence and lends credence to the information the nurse is providing. Often research can provide guidance for surveillance or interventions and give valuable insights. References that are used or referred to should always be properly cited so that the work of researchers is credited. If a presentation is given orally, then the nurse should prepare a list of references. Newsletters, e-mail, or Internet reports and communications should include research highlights or summaries of current studies of interest, with links to online articles provided when possible to encourage people to read the research for themselves and become more knowledgeable about issues related to patients.

Critical reading of research articles

There are a number of steps to critical reading to evaluate research:
- Consider the source of the material. If it is in the popular press, it may have little validity compared to something published in a juried journal.
- Review the author's credentials to determine if a person is an expert in the field of study.
- Determine thesis, or the central claim of the research. It should be clearly stated.
- Examine the organization of the article, whether it is based on a particular theory, and the type of methodology used.
- Review the evidence to determine how it is used to support the main points. Look for statistical evidence and sample size to determine if the findings have wide applicability.
- Evaluate the overall article to determine if the information seems credible and useful and should be communicated to administration and/or staff.

Qualitative and quantitative data

Both qualitative and quantitative data are used for analysis, but the focus is quite different:
- Qualitative data: Data are described verbally or graphically, and the results are subjective, depending upon observers to provide information. Interviews may be used as a tool to gather information, and the researcher's interpretation of data is important. Gathering this type of data can be time-intensive, and it can usually not be generalized to a larger population. This type of information gathering is often useful at the beginning of the design process for data collection.
- Quantitative data: Data are described in terms of numbers within a statistical format. This type of information gathering is done after the design of data collection is outlined, usually in later stages. Tools may include surveys, questionnaires, or other methods of obtaining numerical data. The researcher's role is objective.

Model of integration

Integrating the results of data analysis and research into performance improvement or best practice guidelines varies from one organization to another, depending on the model of integration that the organization uses:
- Organizational: Processes for improvement are identified, and teams or individuals are selected to participate in different areas or departments, reporting to one individual, who monitors progress.
- Functional/coordinated: While staff specialties, such as risk management and quality management, are not integrated, they draw from the same data resources to determine issues related to quality of care and efficiency.
- Functional/integrated: While staff specialties remain, there is cross-training among specialties. A case management approach to individual care is used so that one person follows the progress of a patient through the system and coordinates with the various specialties, such as infection control and quality management.

Synergy model and clinical inquiry

According to the Synergy model, clinical inquiry is a continual process of questioning and evaluating practice in order to provide innovative and outstanding care through application of the results of research and experience. Clinical inquiry requires a desire to acquire new knowledge, openness to accepting advice from mentors and other health and allied professionals, competency in identifying clinical problems, the ability search the literature for research, critical skills to interpret research findings, and the willingness and ability to design and participate in research. Levels of clinical inquiry include:

- Level 1: This nurse recognizes problems and seeks advice, follows industry standards and guidelines, and seeks further knowledge.
- Level 3: This nurse questions industry standards and guidelines as well as current practice and utilizes research and education to improve patient care.
- Level 5: This nurse is able to deviate from industry standards and guidelines when necessary for the individual patients and utilizes literature review and clinical research to gain knowledge, establish new practices, and improve patient care.

Health policy, medical attention, and HIPAA

Health policy – Movement in the direction of primary medical attention and getting prevention earlier; encourages utilization of APRNs. The main elements that control healthcare delivery are payors, insurance companies, providers, and suppliers. Legislation regarding ways to do things and politics is included in this topic.

Medical attention – May be primary health care or managed care. Managed care includes Health Maintenance Organizations (HMO), Preferred Provider Organizations (PPO) and Point of Service (POS) plans.

HIPAA – Health Insurance Portability and Accountability Act of 1996, under Public Law 104-191. This has a goal of better organization and helpfulness in the medical system, which is to be done by regulating the way that electronic communications for administrative and economic information is done. The requirements include particular transaction regulations (including code sets), security and electronic signatures, privacy and particular identifiers that also have utilization permissions for bosses, health plans and people who give medical attention.

Nursing's Agenda for Health Care Reform from ANA (1991)

The Nursing's Agenda for Health Care Reform encourages development of health care which gives patients the ability to get to good medical attention and help without it costing too much, and it encourages continual primary care. It fundamentally asks for vital medical attention to be found for everyone and for there to be a reorganized health care system that centers on patients, well-being and conditions so that they may get medical help in familiar, easy to get to places. It advocates providing for ongoing medical needs and insurance changes so that patients can use their coverage more easily. It asks for organizational assessment on public and private sectors regarding the use of resources, lowering expenses, and getting balanced and even reimbursement for each provider.

Health care reform

Health care reform initiatives are spurring the switch from paper to electronic health records and sharing of health care information among health care providers, increasing the demand for health information technology and people with expertise in informatics. New programs have been developed to focus on wellness with an increased emphasis on cost-effective measures because of increases in health costs. Internal data analysis and research are becoming important means by which to identify waste, institute best practices, and reduce costs. Increasing numbers of people are covered by health plans, even those with preexisting conditions, placing more demand on health care providers for services. There is an increased need for health literacy so that people are better informed about the services available, especially those newly insured. Medicaid costs have increased, resulting in some cutbacks in care. Early transfer from acute care facilities to extended care or home health care is also increasing.

Influential factors on delivery of care

The delivery of care in a system is impacted by a numerous forces:
- Social forces are increasing demand for access to treatment and medical services, both traditional and complementary. As society views equitable medical care as a right, then delivery of care must be available to all.
- Political forces affect medical care as the Federal and state governments increasingly become purchasers of medical care, imposing their guidelines and limitations on the medical system.
- Regulatory forces may be local, state, or Federal and can have a profound effect of delivery of care and services, differing from 1 state or region to another.
- Economic forces, such as managed care or cost-containment committees, try to contain costs to insurers and facilities by controlling access to and duration of treatment, and limiting products. Economic pressure is working to prevent duplication of services in a geographical area, and providers are creating networks to purchase supplies and equipment directly.

Barriers that prevent access to care

There are many barriers that prevent access to care for those with psychiatric and mental health issues:
- Lack of insurance or limited mental health coverage.
- Low income and unemployment.
- Lack of transportation to treatment facilities.
- Language barriers that prevent people from receiving care.
- Inadequate provision of care for children with programs fragmented and often not available, inadequate testing.
- Ethnic minorities with cultural concerns about mental health care or belief systems that preclude their seeking care. Areas with large immigrant populations often lack mental health care tailored to the cultural and language needs of the immigrants.
- Homelessness.
- Lack of mental health care in rural areas.
- Social stigma to mental illness preventing some from seeking care.
- Older adults often overlooked and not assessed for mental health problems.

Poverty
There are a number of issues that impact access to care, but poverty is one of the most significant and can affect care in many ways:
- People may not have health insurance and may not qualify for state medical assistance or may not be aware that they are eligible, so they do not take themselves or children for routine medical visits.
- Practitioners may not accept state medical assistance payments because of low reimbursement rates, leaving people with few options.

- Employers may not allow people to take time off from work during the times that most practices are open to provide care, or people cannot afford to lose income, so most medical care is provided by emergency departments when a crisis arises.
- People may lack automobiles or have insufficient funds for, or access to, public transportation to go to medical visits, especially in more rural areas.

Limits of being low income

Low income often limits access to care. Some people may be eligible for Medicaid, but many of those with psychiatric and mental health problems are ineligible and often lack insurance or the financial resources to pay for care. Free clinics and mental health programs are sometimes available, especially in urban areas, but many people lack access to care or transportation to available care and cannot afford medications. Additionally, rates of depression are higher among those with low income, and depression often prevents people from seeking help. Research indicates that over 40% of those with low income have mental health problems (including depression, panic attacks, and anxiety) or have been diagnosed with a mental disease. Single parents and the unemployed are especially at risk.

Synergy Model in regards to advocacy

Nurse competencies under the Synergy Model include advocacy/moral agency:
- Advocacy is working for the best interests of the patient despite personal values in conflict and assisting patients to have access to appropriate resources.
- Agency is openness and recognition of issues and a willingness to act.
- Moral agency is the ability to recognize needs and take action to influence the outcome of a conflict or decision.

The levels of advocacy/moral agency include:
- Level 1: This nurse works on behalf of the patient, assesses personal values, has awareness of patient's rights and ethical conflicts, and advocates for the patient when consistent with the nurse's personal values.
- Level 3: This nurse advocates for the patient/family, incorporates their values into the care plan even when they differ from the nurse's, and can utilize internal resources to assist patient/family with complex decisions.
- Level 5: This nurse advocates for patient/family despite differences in values and is able to utilize both internal and external resources to help to empower patient/family to make decisions.

Patient advocacy

Patient advocacy is defined as the process of speaking on behalf of a patient to ensure that his or her rights are protected, and that he or she is provided with necessary information and services. The nurse practitioner frequently serves as patient advocate, although physicians, social workers, and other individuals in the health care industry may act on behalf of the patient as well.

Barriers
Patient advocacy is often seen as a moral obligation that the nurse practitioner must fulfill, and is a rewarding part of the nurse practitioner's job; however, patient advocacy can be difficult in certain situations. One barrier to advocacy is a feeling of powerlessness on the part of the nurse

practitioner; sometimes it may feel as if it is the nurse practitioner against the world, especially if the nurse practitioner has no support; lack of support in general is another barrier. A lack of knowledge of the law is another barrier; certain laws may exist, though the nurse practitioner may not be aware of them. If the nurse practitioner and his or her peers are lacking in time, communication, or motivation, advocacy will also prove difficult. Another problem that nurse practitioners frequently encounter is the risk associated with advocacy; included are disagreeing with other nurse practitioners and physicians, and lack of legal support for the advocate.

<u>Facilitators</u>
Perhaps the greatest facilitator of patient advocacy is the nurse practitioner-patient relationship; if a strong relationship exists between the nurse practitioner and the patient, the nurse practitioner will be motivated to perform the duties of advocate. If the patient and nurse practitioner have a strained or limited relationship, advocacy can be difficult. Recognizing the patient's needs is another facilitator, one that goes hand in hand with a good nurse practitioner-patient relationship. If the nurse practitioner feels a sense of responsibility and accountability on behalf of the patient, he or she is more likely to serve as a good patient advocate; conscience is a strong motivator. Another facilitator is if the physician acts as a colleague, instead of a superior; this strengthens the nurse practitioner-physician relationship, and the nurse practitioner feels that he or she can question the physician's judgment instead of constantly deferring. That being said, the greater the knowledge base and skill level of the nurse practitioner, the greater he or she will be as an advocate.

Decreasing the stigma associated with mental illness

Studies have shown that up to a third of Americans relate mental illness to defects of character. Negative beliefs about mental illness persist with people often fearing those who are mentally ill. Effective methods to decrease the stigma associated with mental illness include:
- Educating people about mental illness: People need to know factual information, including about levels of violence associated with those who are mentally ill since this is a pervasive concern. People should be advised of the incidence of mental illness and available treatments.
- Using words carefully: Healthcare providers and others should choose words carefully, avoiding words such as "nuts" and "crazy," and remembering to put the person first: "person with schizophrenia" rather than "schizophrenic."
- Providing support services: Helping the mentally ill finds places to live and providing other necessary services may help to reduce substance abuse and homelessness, which increase stigma.
- Increasing contact: Integrating those with mental illness into the community through job placement and housing helps others to become more familiar with those who are mentally ill.

Impact of social, political, regulatory, and economic forces on delivery of care

The delivery of care is impacted by a numerous forces:
- Social forces are increasing demand for access to treatment and medical services, both traditional and complementary. As society views equitable medical care as a right, then delivery of care must be available to all.

- Political forces affect medical care as the Federal and state governments increasingly become purchasers of medical care, imposing their guidelines and limitations on the medical system.
- Regulatory forces may be local, state, or Federal and can have a profound effect of delivery of care and services, differing from one state or region to another.
- Economic forces, such as managed care or cost-containment committees, try to contain costs to insurers and facilities by controlling access to and duration of treatment, and limiting products. Economic pressure is working to prevent duplication of services in a geographical area, and providers are creating networks to purchase supplies and equipment directly.

ANA's definition of nursing

The ANA defines nursing as "the protection, promotion, and optimization of health and abilities, prevention of illness and injury, alleviation of suffering through the diagnosis and treatment of human response, and advocacy in the care of individuals, families, communities, and populations."

HIPAA

In 1996, Congress passed the Health Insurance Portability and Accountability Act (HIPAA), which includes a number of provisions that aim to improve the portability of health information records. The Department of Health and Human Services was charged with establishing national healthcare standards for storage and transfer of electronic healthcare information to improve the exchange of information from 1 insurance company/physician to another. In the past, a patient's complete record would be stored and others could access these records easily. Strides are being made toward improving the privacy of the patient, however standardization has not yet occurred and different electronic storage systems are often incompatible. HIPAA requires that healthcare providers use a National Provider Identifier (NPI), which is a 10-digit number. HIPAA includes strong provisions to protect the privacy of the individual in order to prevent abuse and misuse of records.

Confidentiality

Confidentiality is the obligation that is present in a professional-patient relationship. Nurse practitioners are under an obligation to protect the information they possess concerning the patient and family. Care should be taken to safeguard that information and provide the privacy that the patient deserves. This is accomplished through the use of required passwords when the family calls for information about the patient and through the limitation of who is allowed to visit. The nurse practitioner should not assume that family members can be apprised of an older adult's health information without that person's consent. There may be times when confidentiality must be broken to save the life of a patient, but those circumstances are rare. The nurse practitioner must make all efforts to safeguard patient records and identification. Computerized record keeping should be done in such a way that the screen is not visible to others, and paper records must be secured.

Need-to-know information

Patients have a right to expect that when they divulge personal information to a nurse practitioner that only those with a need to know will be provided this information. When nurse practitioners must document care, they must be sensitive to the information that they put into the written record or report because many people have access to these records. If the information is health-related, then the practitioner is obligated to record this and should tell the patient. Need-to-know issues also relate to the patient's need to know about care and prognosis. Patients may be overwhelmed by information or they may be cognitively impaired or confused. Older adults and families should be asked how much information they want. Some patients/families want to know all of the details, including treatment options and expected outcomes. Others want only the basic information or don't want to discuss health issues at all.

Computer system standards

The Joint Commission has described the need for computer system standards in the following areas:
- Access to databases that are located outside the organization and used to compare information, need to be supported and secured.
- Patient confidentiality related to personal health information (PHI) and data security must be ensured.
- Knowledge-based systems should be developed and promoted to allow resident organizational expertise to be used throughout the organization.
- A means to link physician information systems while protecting patient privacy and data security.
- Projects that are designed to achieve quality improvements should be supported.
- Data integrity and overall system security must be ensured.
- Procedural controls that are currently in place for documentation should be integrated into the new computerized standards.
- A regular assessment of needs and system capacity for growth should be supported.

Important factors for information systems

The Joint Commission outlined factors it believes are important for information standards:
- Measures must be adopted that are designed to protect an individual's personal health information. This may be accomplished by limiting access to information based on a user's need to know, having strict policies regarding the removal of records, and making sure data is physically and electronically safeguarded.
- A national standard for data entry should be created and followed. All users should be trained both in system use and information management. Educational courses may include lectures on how information that is entered into a computer system is transformed into data that can later be used to support decision-making and perform statistical analysis.
- All information should be available both on the computer and in print form.

Electronic medical records and electronic health records

Although many in healthcare use the terms electronic medical record (EMR) and electronic health record (EHR) interchangeably, there are major distinctions between the two. The electronic medical record is created by a hospital or other health care delivery organization (CDO). The CDO owns the information in the EMR. The EMR consists of clinical documentation, orders, medications, treatments, and other clinical decision support, and is a legal record. The EHR includes information from EMRs, likely from multiple health care delivery organizations. The EHR relies on the information from the EMR to complete it. The EHR is owned by the patient and stakeholders, which could include the government, insurance companies, and healthcare providers among others. Important to the EMR is using controlled medical vocabulary so that information will be

- 66 -

comparable among providers and other interested stakeholders. Currently in the United States the use of EHRs is limited, mostly due to many healthcare delivery organizations not having an established EMR using decided predetermined standards. There may soon be an increase in the number of organizations using EMRs with standardized language conducive to EHRs, as organizations now receive financial incentives to install EMR and EHR systems from health care reform.

The Healthcare Information and Management Systems Society (HIMSS) define the electronic health record (EHR) as a "secure, real-time, point-of-care, patient-centric information resource for clinicians." HIMSS has also published a series of guidelines for EHR known as the HIMSS Electronic Health Record Definitional Model. According to the model, the EHR should record and manage information for both the short- and long-term. The EHR should be the healthcare professional's main resource when taking care of patients. Evidence-based care can be planned using the EHR on both the individual and community level. Another important job of the EHR is its use in continuous quality improvement, performance management, risk management, utilization review, and resource planning. The EHR aids in the billing process as well. Finally, the EHR is a boon to evidence-based research, clinical research, and public health reporting. Since it is computerized, clinicians are assured that the EHR information is up to date and relevant for patients and research protocols.

Goals of mental health education

Mental health education is the imparting of mental health knowledge to clients and their families. According to Walker and Price-Hoskins (1992), the goals of mental health education include:
- Offering information about the illness and appropriate interventions.
- Helping people recognize symptoms.
- Teaching people when and how to intervene for themselves.
- Offering relief from guilt and blame.
- Clarifying family expectations.
- Instilling confidence that change can occur.
- Developing perspective and balance.

Methods used for education include lecture, discussion, modeling, observation, experiential (role playing and behavioral rehearsal), coaching, audiovisual presentations, and self-instruction (such as keeping a diary). Guidelines for teaching adult learners include: assessing the client's knowledge base; increasing the awareness for self-learning; encouraging self-direction; encouraging the application of what has been learned; using modes of learning most useful to client; and repeating, changing, and combining teaching methods and modes as needed.

Readiness to learn

The patient/family's readiness to learn should be assessed because if they are not ready, instruction is of little value. Often readiness is indicated when the patient/family asks questions or shows an interest in procedures. There are a number of factors related to readiness to learn:
- Physical factors: There are a number of physical factors than can affect ability. Manual dexterity may be required to complete a task, and this varies by age and condition. Hearing or vision deficits may impact ability. Complex tasks may be too difficult for some because of weakness or cognitive impairment, and modifications of the environment may be needed. Health status, age, and gender may all impact the ability to learn.

- Experience: People's experience with learning can vary widely and is affected by their ability to cope with changes, their personal goals, motivation to learn, and cultural background. People may have widely divergent ideas about what constitutes illness and/or treatment. Lack of English skills may make learning difficult and prevent people from asking questions.
- Mental/emotional status: The support system and motivation may impact readiness. Anxiety, fear, or depression about the patient's condition can make learning very difficult because the patient/family cannot focus on learning, so the nurse practitioner must spend time to reassure the patient/family and wait until they are emotionally more receptive.
- Knowledge/education: The knowledge base of the patient/family, their cognitive ability, and their learning styles all affect their readiness to learn. The nurse should always begin by assessing what knowledge the patient/family already have about their disease, condition, or treatment and then build from that base. People with little medical experience may lack knowledge of basic medical terminology, interfering with their ability and readiness to learn.

Approaches to teaching

There are many approaches to teaching, and the nurse practitioner may need to prepare, present, and coordinate a wide range of educational workshops, lectures, discussions, and one-on-one instructions on any chosen topic. All of the following types of classes will be needed, depending upon the purpose and material:
- Educational workshops are usually conducted with small groups, allowing for maximal participation, and are especially good for demonstrations and practice sessions.
- Lectures are often used for more academic or detailed information that may include questions and answers, but limit discussion. An effective lecture should include some audiovisual support.
- Discussions are best with small groups so that people can actively participate. This is a good for problem solving.
- One-on-one instruction is especially helpful for targeted instruction in procedures for individuals.
- Computer/Internet modules are good for independent learners.

Participants should be asked to evaluate the presentations in the forms of surveys or suggestions, but ultimately the program is evaluated in terms of patient outcomes.

Readability

Studies have indicated that learning is more effective if oral presentations and/or demonstrations are supplemented with reading materials, such as handouts. Readability (the grade level of material) is a concern because many patients and families may have limited English skills or low literacy, and it can be difficult for the nurse to assess people's reading level. The average American reads effectively at the sixth to eighth grade level (regardless of education achieved), but many health education materials have a much higher readability level. Additionally, research indicates that even people with much higher reading skills learn medical and health information most effectively when the material is presented at the sixth to eighth grade readability level. Therefore, patient education materials (and consent forms) should not be written at higher than sixth to eighth grade level. Readability index calculators are available on the Internet to give an approximation of grade level and difficulty for those preparing materials without expertise in teaching reading.

Bloom's taxonomy and 3 types of learning

Bloom's taxonomy outlines behaviors that are necessary for learning, and this can apply to health care. The theory describes 3 types of learning:

- Cognitive: (Learning and gaining intellectual skills to master 6 categories of effective learning.)
  - o Knowledge
  - o Comprehension
  - o Application
  - o Analysis
  - o Synthesis
  - o Evaluation.
- Affective: (Recognizing 5 categories of feelings and values from simple to complex. This is slower to achieve than cognitive learning.)
  - o Receiving phenomena: Accepting the need to learn.
  - o Responding to phenomena: Taking active part in care.
  - o Valuing: Understanding value of becoming independent in care.
  - o Organizing values: Understanding how surgery/treatment has improved life.
  - o Internalizing values: Accepting condition as part of life, being consistent and self-reliant.
- Psychomotor: (Mastering 6 motor skills necessary for independence. This follows a progression from simple to complex.)
  - o Perception: Uses sensory information to learn tasks.
  - o Set: Shows willingness to perform tasks. Guided response: Follows directions. Mechanism: Does specific tasks.
  - o Complex overt response: Displays competence in self-care.
  - o Adaptation: Modifies procedures as needed.
  - o Origination: Creatively deals with problems.

Adult learning styles

Not all people are aware of their preferred learning style. A range of teaching materials/methods that relates to all 3 learning preferences—visual, auditory, kinesthetic—(and age-appropriate) should be available. Part of assessment for teaching involves choosing the right approach based on observation and feedback. Often presenting learners with different options gives a clue to their preferred learning style. Some people have a combined learning style:

Visual learners	Learn best by seeing and reading: • Provide written directions, picture guides, or demonstrate procedures. • Use charts and diagrams. • Provide photos, videos.

Auditory learners	Learn best by listening and talking:
	• Explain procedures while demonstrating and have learner repeat.
	• Plan extra time to discuss and answer questions.
	• Provide audiotapes.
Kinesthetic learners	Learn best by handling, doing, and practicing:
	• Provide hands-on experience throughout teaching.
	• Encourage handling of supplies/equipment.
	• Allow learner to demonstrate.
	• Minimize instructions and allow person to explore equipment and procedures.

Teaching strategies for adult learners

Adults have a wealth of life and/or employment experiences. Their attitudes toward education may vary considerably. There are, however, some principles of adult learning and typical characteristics of adult learners that an instructor should consider when planning strategies for teaching parents, families, or staff:

Practical and goal-oriented	Provide overviews or summaries and examples. Use collaborative discussions with problem-solving exercises. Remain organized with the goal in mind.
Self-directed	Provide active involvement, asking for input. Allow different options toward achieving the goal. Give them responsibilities.
Knowledgeable	Show respect for their life experiences/education. Validate their knowledge and ask for feedback. Relate new material to information with which they are familiar.
Relevancy-oriented	Explain how information will be applied. Clearly identify objectives.
Motivated	Provide certificates of achievement or some type of recognition for achievement

Teaching older adults

There are a number of strategies that facilitate teaching older adults:
- Spend a little time getting to know the patient so that he/she is more relaxed and receptive to learning.
- Determine what information is critical for the patient to learn and what is non-essential.
- Evaluate the patient's learning style and previous knowledge about the topic.
- Plan for ample time for each session of instruction and plan the probable number of sessions to determine how much instruction is needed for each session. Ensure that sessions are presented in a closely-spaced manner to reinforce learning.
- Provide the patient ample time to practice.
- Allow the patient to guide the pace of the session as much as possible and encourage feedback.
- Prepare age-appropriate handouts at accessible reading level and with large-size font.
- Provide materials (pencil, paper) in case the patient wants to make notes.
- Be supportive, patient, and enthusiastic.

Teaching and learning for children ages 6 to 11

From ages 6 to 11, children vary widely in physical maturity, but they have increasing control of fine and gross motor skills, are receptive to learning, can question, and reason. Thinking remains literal rather than abstract. Concentration improves with age, and older children have a better understanding of their body and body systems. They are used to structured education. Children interact with peers and fear being different or ill. Teaching is aimed at the child with the parents as support (especially in later childhood). Some techniques commonly used to teach children include:

- Allow children to assume responsibility for much of their care.
- Limit teaching to about 30 minutes and allow time for the child to absorb and study material.
- Provide age-specific materials, such as Kid Cards (medicine information cards).
- Use a variety of teaching materials, including pictures, diagrams, and illustrations.
- Use analogies (A CT is like a giant camera).
- Use one-on-one or group instruction as appropriate.
- Tell children about treatments/procedures in advance.
- Provide support and encourage questions and participation.

Kid Cards

One of the challenges to facilitating learning in children is to teach them about their medications. Kid Cards are medicine information cards that present important details about the medication in language that is age-appropriate and often with pictures or illustrations. Information on a Kid Card may include:

Methylphenidate
This medicine is also called Ritalin LA®.

Why am I taking Ritalin?
- You have to take this medicine so you can think better.
- It helps you to relax and listen better to others.

How do I take Ritalin?
- It is a capsule (about the size of a peanut M&M).
- You need to take 1 capsule each morning with breakfast. You can open the capsule and sprinkle the medicine on applesauce, but don't chew up the capsule.

What might happen if I take Ritalin?
- Most kids don't have any bad effects from taking Ritalin.

If you get a rash, start itching, have stomach pain, feel nervous, can't sleep, feel "funny," or have a headache, tell your mom right away so she can call the doctor.

Play to facilitate learning

Play can be a useful tool to help children deal with physical and emotional problems related to their illness. Allowing children to play with medical equipment under supervision can allay some of their fears and help them to understand. Needle play, in which the child gives "shots" to a doll (with safe plastic syringes) can help them to express feelings about blood draws or injections. Providing dolls and puppets and engaging in play may encourage the child to express anxiety and fear through "talking" for the toy. There are a number of specialty dolls, such as dolls with removable parts to show internal organs and Shadow Buddies®, which are dolls that are commercially available (custom-made) to show the effects of different illnesses or surgeries. For example, a doll with thinning hair may show the effects of chemotherapy. Other dolls have stomas and colostomy bags. Drawing also may encourage the child to express feelings.

Teaching and learning for adolescents

Adolescents vary widely in both physical and emotional maturity; they have good reasoning and abstract thinking skills, understand cause and effect, and have good motor skills, but may engage in risk-taking behaviors and may have difficulty dealing with illness and poor compliance with treatments. They are very conscious of their body image and have a strong need to belong to a peer group, often rebelling against authority. They wish to be independent and need privacy and confidentiality. Teaching is aimed at allowing the adolescent to be independent in care:
- Use one-on-one (for confidential teaching) or peer group instruction/discussion as appropriate.
- Supplement instruction with audiovisual materials, computer-generated instruction, models, diagrams, illustrations, and written instructions, focusing on learning style and learning preferences.
- Allow the adolescent to maintain as much control over learning as possible.
- Provide options from which the adolescent can choose.
- Be patient, respectful, and tactful.
- Provide reasons for everything.
- Avoid conflict and direct confrontation, but suggest alternatives.

Joint Commission

The Joint Commission has established leadership standards that apply to healthcare organizations and help to establish management's lines of authority and accountability. Under these standards, leadership comprises the governing body, the chief executive office and senior managers, department leaders, leaders (both elected and appointed) of staff or departments, and the nurse executive and other nurse leaders. The governing body is ultimately responsible for all patient care rendered by all types of practitioners (physicians, nurses, laboratory staff, support staff, etc) within and under the jurisdiction of the organization, so this governing body must clearly outline the line of authority and accountability for others in management positions. At each level of management, performance standards and performance measurements should be established so that accountability becomes transparent based on data that can be used to drive changes when needed and to bring about improved outcomes.

Accreditation

Accreditation is a primary requirement for organization because it establishes that the organization is committed to standards based on evaluation. General accreditation is usually done by the following:
- The Joint Commission accredits more than 20,000 healthcare programs, both nationally and internationally, and is the primary accrediting agency in the United States, so accreditation

by the Joint Commission indicates a commitment to improving care and provides information about compliance with core measures.
- The Healthcare Facilities Accreditation Program of the American Osteopathic Association also accredits many healthcare programs, including acute care, ambulatory care, rehabilitation and substance abuse centers, behavioral care centers, and critical access hospitals, and also provides guidelines for patient safety initiatives as well as reports of common deficiencies.

A healthcare organization may also seek to become accredited by agencies with a narrower focus to demonstrate excellence in that area, such as the Intersocietal Commission for the Accreditation of Echocardiography Laboratories (ICAEL). Leadership and staff must determine what type of accreditation is most appropriate based on the programs offered and the commitment to improving standards.

Consumer-focused health care

Consumer-focused health care recognizes that the needs of the patient are central to delivery of care and that provision of care should try to match the expectations of the patient. With the Internet, patients have easy access to much more medical information than previously, and as patients become better informed, they expect a greater role in their own healthcare decisions and better quality care at lower prices. A primary component of consumer-focused health care is evaluating customer satisfaction and utilizing continuous quality improvement methods to improve service. The needs of the patient are viewed holistically, so that all healthcare needs are met, ranging from housing to medical treatment. The nurse practitioner must be an advocate for the patient, assessing patients' expectations and implementing changes to assure that the needs are met. Because patients often fail to express their dissatisfaction directly to healthcare providers, the nurse should ask patients directly if they have concerns.

Case management

One model for managing patient care is to use a case manager. The case manager is responsible for identifying needs of the patient, finding resources, linking the patient with needed services both within a mental health facility and in the community, and monitoring the patient. Within an acute, sub-acute, or skilled nursing facility, the case manager may chair the interdisciplinary team to ensure that the needs of the patient are communicated and that all members of the team are focused on similar goals. As the patient moves back into the community, the case manager needs to consider the social support services (home health care, transportation, meals-on-wheels, etc) that are needed for the person to remain as independent as possible and to function safely. The case manager supervises and manages all aspects of care to ensure continuity.

Need for adequate housing

The need for adequate housing is an ongoing problem with psychiatric patients. Many of these patients are homeless and once released from inpatient care services do not have anywhere to live and may be estranged from family, leaving them with no support system. A safe and affordable option is vital to the success of their treatment. Many mental health patients have a relapse of their mental illness, suffer medical illness, incarceration, or abuse by others. The most common housing available includes group homes, such as personal care homes or board-and-care homes, therapeutic foster care, and supervised apartments. Many of these provide some type of rehabilitation and/or support services such as group therapy, job training, and counseling to help the patient make the transition from the treatment facility to the home environment and to learn to manage self-care.

Therapeutic foster care homes and supervised apartments

Therapeutic foster care provides for the patient in a home setting with a family that is trained to care for high-need patients. This training includes medication education, crisis management, and disease education. The foster family supervises all aspects of the patient's care and incorporates the patient into the structure of the home. Many times the patient will share household work and may attend daytime care programs. This level of care is available for both children and adults. Supervised apartments provide residents with individual apartments. Residents may either live alone or share the apartment with a roommate. They are responsible for the upkeep of the apartment and are independent in their self-care needs. The apartment is supervised by staff members that regularly check on the residents to ensure that they are doing well and following prescribed medication regimes.

Personal care homes and board-and-care homes

Personal care homes, also called residential care facilities, are located in homes in residential communities. These homes can usually provide supervised care for up to approximately 10 individuals, depending on licensure. Services often include: supervising medication regimens, providing for transportation needs, serving meals, and assisting with activities of daily living. Many of the residents are elderly or suffer mild intellectual disability or psychiatric illness. Board-and-care homes are similar to personal care homes; however, there is little assistance with activities of daily living although meals are usually provided. Many of the residents can provide their own self-care with little supervision. Board-and-care homes are usually larger in size and accommodate up to 150 individuals. Both types of residential services are licensed by the state.

Medicare

Medicare, provides payment to private healthcare providers, such as physicians and hospitals, but limits reimbursement. Physicians receive 80% of usual, customary, and reasonable (UCR) fees if they accept Medicare assignment. If they do not, they can charge up to 115% of what Medicare allows. Patients are responsible for the remaining 20% or up to 115% if the physicians do not accept Medicare. Parts include:
- Medicare A: Hospital insurance covers acute hospital, limited nursing home care, and/or home health care, as well as hospice care for the terminally ill. There is no premium for this part.
- Medicare B: Medical insurance covers physicians, nurse practitioners, laboratory, physical, and occupational therapy. Patients must pay an annual deductible as well as a monthly payment.
- Medicare D: Prescription drug plan covers part of the costs of prescription drugs at participating pharmacies. It is administered by private insurance companies, so monthly costs and benefits vary somewhat.

Medicaid

Medicaid is a combined federal and state welfare program authorized by Title XIX of the Social Security Act and regulated by the Centers for Medicare and Medicaid Services (CMS) to assist low-income individuals with payment for medical care. This program provides assistance for all ages, including children. Older adults receiving supplemental security income (SSI) are eligible, as are others who meet state eligibility requirements. The Medicaid programs are administered by the individual states, which establish eligibility and reimbursement guidelines, so benefits vary considerably from 1 state to another. Older adults with Medicare are eligible for Medicaid as a secondary insurance. Expenses that may be covered for adults include inpatient and outpatient hospital services, physician payments, nursing home care, home health care, and laboratory and radiation services. Adults who are legal resident aliens are ineligible for Medicaid for 5 years after attaining legal resident status. Some states pay for preventive services, such as home and community-based programs aimed at reducing the need for hospitalization.

EPO, HMO, PPO, and POS

There are a number of different models for managed care to provide healthcare services:
- Exclusive provider organization (EPO): Healthcare providers provide services at discounted rates to those enrolled in a service. Some providers may be prohibited from caring for those not enrolled and enrollees are only reimbursed for care within the network.
- Health maintenance organization (HMO): With an HMO, there is a prepaid contract between healthcare providers, payors, and enrollees for specified services in a specified time period, provided by a list of providers, usually representing a variety of specialties.
- Preferred provider organizations: (PPO): This involves healthcare providers who have agreed to be part of a network providing services to an enrolled group at reduced rates of reimbursement. Care received outside of the network is usually only partially covered.
- Point-of-service plans (POS): This is a combination HMO and PPO structure so that people can receive service in the network but can opt to seek treatment outside the network in some situations.

Tricare

Tricare is the healthcare program serving active military, retired military, and their spouses and dependents. Tricare provides a number of different plans, depending upon location and eligibility. For those with Medicare, Tricare becomes the secondary insurer. If patients choose to opt out of Medicare (such as those with no insurance or private insurance), Tricare pays the amount equivalent to a secondary insurer (20% of allowable), and the patient is responsible for the rest. By law, all other insurances must pay before Tricare. Patients may access care at military treatment facilities (MTF) on a space-available basis, but must enroll in Tricare Plus to receive primary care at MTFs. Those eligible for both Tricare and Veterans Affairs (VA) programs may receive care at VA medical facilities, if the service is covered under Tricare and the facility is part of the Tricare network; however, the VA cannot bill Medicare so costs not covered by Tricare must be paid by the patient even if the patient has Medicare coverage.

Billing codes

In order to be reimbursed by insurance companies and Medicare or Medicaid, the nurse practitioner must provide appropriate billing codes. Reimbursement may require use of different codes. Most healthcare providers use standard forms with checklists of diagnosis and appropriate coding. In many cases, denial of services relates to incorrect coding.

Coding systems include:

- International Classification of Disease (ICD): Developed by the World Health Organization (WHO) and used to code for diagnosis.
- Diagnostic-related group (DRG): Used to classify a disorder according to diagnosis and treatment.
- Current procedural terminology (CPT): Developed by the American Medical Society and used to define those licensed to provide services and to describe medical treatments and procedures.
- Universal billing (UB): Used to describe hospital services, including demographic information, diagnostic and treatment codes, and charges for services. UB-04 is the current version.

Older Americans Act/Ombudsman

The Older Americans Act (OAA) (Title III) of 1965 (amended in 2006) provides improved access to services for older adults and Native Americans, including community services (meals, transportation, home health care, adult day care, legal assistance, and home repair). The OAA provides funding to local area agencies on aging (AAA) or state or tribal agencies, which administer funding. These local agencies can assess community needs and contract for services. One of the programs commonly supported with funds from the OAA is meals-on-wheels. Low cost adult day care is also offered in some communities. The OAA includes the National Family Caregivers Support Act, which provides services for caregivers of older adults. The OAA also provides grants for programs that combat violence against older adults and others to provide computer training for older adults. Additionally, the OAA mandates that each state have an ombudsman program. Ombudsmen provide services to residents of nursing homes and other facilities to insure that care meets state standards.

OBRA

The Omnibus Budget Reconciliation Act (OBRA) of 1987 contains the 1990 Nursing Home Reform Amendments (NHRA). These amendments establish guidelines for nursing facilities (such as long-term care facilities). Provisions include:

- Complete physical and mental assessment of each patient on admission, annually, and with change of condition.
- Requirement for 24-hour nursing care with registered nurses (RNs) on duty for at least 1 shift.
- Nurse aide training is mandated as well as regular inservice and state registry of trained/qualified aides.
- Rehabilitative services must be available.
- Physicians/physician's assistant/nurse practitioner must visit every 30 days for the first 3 months and then every 90 days.
- Outlawing/discouraging Medicaid discrimination.
- Requirement for independent monitoring of psychopharmacologic drugs.
- Recognition of patients' rights.
- Survey protocols to assess patient care and patient outcomes.
- State sanctions to enforce nursing home regulations.

EMTALA

The Emergency Medical Treatment and Active Labor Act (EMTALA) is designed to prevent patient "dumping" from emergency departments (EDs) and is an issue of concern for risk management, requiring staff training for compliance: EMTALA guidelines concerning the transfer of an ED patient include:

- Transfers from the ED may be intrahospital or to another facility.
- Stabilization of the patient with emergency conditions or active labor must be done in the ED prior to transfer, and initial screening must be given prior to inquiring about insurance or ability to pay.
- Stabilization requires treatment for emergency conditions and reasonable belief that, although the emergency condition may not be completely resolved, the patient's condition will not deteriorate during transfer.
- Women in the ED in active labor should deliver both the child and placenta before transfer.
- The receiving department or facility should be capable of treating the patient and dealing with complications that might occur.
- Transfer to another facility is indicated if the patient requires specialized services not available intrahospital, such as to burn centers.

Mental Health Parity Act

The Mental Health Parity Act (1996) is a law that applies to large group health plans. This act is designed as a protection for individuals with mental disabilities and disorders. The Mental Health Parity Act mandates equal annual and lifetime dollar benefits for mental health treatment compared to that available for medical and surgical treatments. This act only applies to the financial responsibility of the plan and does allow for other restrictions within the plan, such as a limit on the number of visits to a mental health professional and access to network providers only. Substance abuse and chemical dependency are not covered by the law. The exact specifications vary by plan and the provisions of the Mental Health Parity Act do not apply to small group health plans.

School resources

School resources vary widely. Most colleges and universities provide mental health services to students. Some have mental health clinics or other counselling services available, and these services can provide valuable support for students with psychiatric or mental health concerns. K-12 schools are more limited in the mental health services that they provide. In some cases, the school nurse or academic counselors may provide some mental health counselling or referrals, but mental health professionals are usually not available on site. Children who are receiving mental health care and/or medications may need support in the school environment, so the nurse practitioner and family may need to discuss the needs with the school administration to determine what services the school is able to provide. *SchoolMentalHealth.org*, a feature of the Baltimore School Mental Health Technical Assistance and Training Initiative, provides resources for students, healthcare providers, educators, and educators with protocols for management of different types of behavioral problems, such as anger management.

Resource utilization

Resource utilization refers to the consideration of all factors related to the planning and delivery of quality patient care. Resources may be allotted to the physical environment for building or remodeling, staffing, equipment, literature, training, and outreach programs. Utilization review requires consideration of patient safety, treatment effectiveness, and cost of care. The patient should receive mental health care that meets all of the factors. The care should be safe, effective, and affordable for each individual patient. Treatment decisions should take into consideration rising healthcare costs and how to maximize the use of resources while continuing to provide quality patient care. The goal of resource utilization is to provide quality, cost-effective care, while utilizing the best-qualified staff and appropriate resources.

Continuum of care

The continuum of care can move from inpatient treatments to various outpatient treatments and support systems, including in-home family treatment. Treatment may begin with acute crisis intervention and stabilization in the hospital setting, may then move to partial hospitalization allowing for the patient to leave for periods of time or go home at night, and finally to return home fulltime. This allows for varying levels of intensity throughout the patient treatment program and allows for treatment to be coordinated in many different environmental settings, care levels, by different healthcare providers, and by a variety of different services. This continuum of care occurs over a long period of time and includes the involvement of many different services. Its purpose is to meet the comprehensive needs of the patient through the coordination of interdisciplinary care and services. Outpatient treatment programs as well as supportive employment programs also participate in the provision of the continuum of care.

SAMHSA and NMHIC

The Substance Abuse and Mental Health Services Administration's (SAMHSA's) National Mental Health Information Center (NMHIC) provides information about opportunities for grants and application forms as well as a number of resources for mental health professionals. SAMSHA (http://www.samhsa.gov/index.aspx) provides grants in a wide range of areas, including supportive housing, suicide prevention, family intervention, jail diversion, traumatic stress, and substance abuse prevention. The NMHIC provides fact sheets and brochures, which can be ordered for distribution, on all aspects of mental illness. Training guides are also available free of charge. NMHIC also provides state resource guides for each state. Many fact sheet and reports are available for download directly from the website. SAMHSA provides a newsroom that lists all press announcements, including information about available grants and recent awards.

NAMI

The National Alliance on Mental Illness (NAMI) is an invaluable community resource for those with mental illness and their families. Programs include:
- Family-to-Family: Free 12-week course intended to help family members or caregivers of those with severe psychiatric disorders (such as schizophrenia or bipolar disorder).
- In Our Own Voice: People living with mental illness speak about their experiences and recovery.
- NAMI Connection: Weekly support groups for those with mental illness.
- Parents and Teachers as Allies: Two-hour inservice program for teachers about early signs of mental illness, interventions, and dealing with families.
- Peer-to-Peer: Nine 2-hour courses taught by trained mentors with a history of mental illness, teaching participants to better manage their mental illness and avoid relapses.

- NAMI Provider Education: Ten-week course taught by a panel of 5 (2 family members, 2 mental health patients, and a mental health professional) for staff working directly with people with mental illness.

Home meal delivery programs

Home meal delivery programs (such as Meals-on-Wheels) provide nutritious meals for homebound older adults or others who are physically or mentally disabled. The programs usually serve meals 5-7 days a week with home delivery, often by volunteers. Meals are usually low cost ($2-5 per meal) but this varies with program. Most programs deliver 1 hot meal a day and may provide food for 1 or 2 other meals (such as a sandwich for dinner and cold cereal for breakfast the next day). Requirements and age restrictions vary with some primarily serving those ≥60 and others ≥65. People with temporary disabilities may be restricted in length of service. Some programs are intended for those with low incomes but others do not have income restrictions. Most programs provide little choice in menu but may offer low-fat, low-salt, or low-carbohydrate diets. Many home meal delivery programs have waiting lists because the need outpaces the number of programs.

Independent Practice Competencies

Standards of advance practice

The nurse practitioner (NP) must practice within the standards of advance practice and the individual's scope of practice, which is directly related to the individual's educational preparation and certification. A NP must have 2 types of licenses/certificates: a registered nurse (RN) license and an advanced practice certificate. Advance practice nurses are those who have completed additional education in an accredited nursing program (usually at a Master's level) and have received certification with a national certifying organization, such as the American Nurse's Credentialing Center. The NP must function legally under the Nurse Practice Act of the state in which the person resides. In some cases, a NP license/certification in 1 state is automatically recognized in other states through the Compact agreement, but advance practice nurses are often excluded from these agreements. Educational experience and scope of practice must relate to patient population in terms of age, disease, diagnosis, and treatment.

The specific responsibilities involved in standards of advance practice include:
- Documentation: The nurse practitioner (NP) keeps accurate, legal, and legible records and also maintains patient confidentiality. The NP ensures that the patient signs a release before providing medical records to other parties.
- Patient advocacy: The NP advocates for the individual patient in the process of care but also advocates for patients at the state and national level in order to facilitate patient access to care and improve the quality of care.
- Continuous quality improvement: The NP recognizes the need for constant learning, evaluation, and reevaluation and participates in quality review, continuing education while maintaining certification, and utilizing clinical guidelines and standards of care.
- Research and education: The NP initiates, participates in, and utilizes the results of research in clinical practice.

Nursing practice acts

See the NCSBN Web site to find the complete list of state practice acts (not for every state, but 31 states are included): http://www.ncsbn.org. An authorizing board of nursing is available in every state to lead statutes with regard to licenses for an RN. They have responsibility for how titles are used, scope of work, and how to handle discipline cases. Nurse practice acts come out of statutory law.

Advanced practice registered nursing

According to the NCSBN, advanced practice registered nursing (APRN) is acting as a nurse with a foundation on information and proficiency that was obtained in basic nursing school. This nurse has a license to be an RN and has completed and received a diploma from graduate school in an APRN program that has been accredited from a nationwide accrediting body. This nurse has up-to-date certification from a nationwide certification board to work in the proper APRN area. Being an APRN defines the nurse as someone that has more responsibility, which may or may not come with more pay or gain for the nurse.

Some responsibilities include:
- Give professional education and leadership.
- Handle patient and medical center leadership.
- Support the patient and local area by keeping the ideal concerns for the patient or community.
- Assess reactions of involvement and how well medical routines are working.
- Be in touch with and act together with patients, patient relatives, and colleagues.
- Employ research; get and use new information and equipment.
- Educate others regarding APRN.

Scope of practice

It is dependent on each state and what the APRN in this position can do beneath the Nurse Practice Act for that state. The scope gives guidelines instead of particular directives. There is a big range, depending on the state. Many times the scope is founded on what is allowed legally both in the state and in the nation. The initial Scope of Practice for PNPs occurred in 1983 by the National Association of Pediatric Nurse Practitioners. This has been updated in 1990 and in 2000. Scope is always changing and improving.

Responsibilities

Responsibilities of the advanced practice registered nurse (APRN) include but are not limited to the following:
- Evaluate the patient, produce and assess information; comprehend higher nursing practice in action at this rank.
- Assess many kinds of information; find differential diagnosis; determine proper medical care.
- Without supervision, determine how to handle difficult patient issues.
- Create a way to identify the condition, create objectives for the patient's medical management, and stipulate the medical routine or plan.
- Identify, set the routine for medical management, oversee, and give out the medical plan. This includes medicine and drugs as appropriate that fall inside of the APRN's area.
- Handle the patient's bodily and mental condition.
- Make sure there is protected and pertinent nursing being done, whether direct or indirect with regard to the patient.
- Keep protected and beneficial surroundings.

Credentials

Credentials for APRN:
- Make sure there is answerability and conscientiousness for proficient work.
- Authenticates that the practioner has received the correct instruction, has a license, and is certified.
- Compulsory to make sure that the local and national laws are followed. Recognizes the furthered scope for the APRN.
- Allows for needed ways for patients to make a grievance.
- Allows for responsibility for the community by making sure standards of practice are met.
- Debates between the State boards of Nursing and different education accrediting organizations were more heated in the 1990s due to more NP programs coming available.
- National task force with regard to the excellence of NP schools met in 1995. Many organizations were present.
- The government does not have a hand in credentialing.

- Credentials may be obtained through an AACN-acknowledged certifying body.

<u>Certification and writing prescriptions</u>
The government has no responsibility for certification. An agency or group verifies that the nurse has a license and has finished specific, set-forth standards as must be met in the particular area of expertise. It might be necessary to receive a state license or reimbursement. It is necessary to become an APRN in certain states. NPs and Certified Nurse-Midwives (CNM) have had the ability to write certain prescriptions since the mid-1970s. Since 1998, every state allows a degree of ability to write prescriptions. It is necessary that pharmacology instruction be included in the master's degree; the APRN has to get continued instruction to keep the authority to write prescriptions. Certain guidelines differ between the states. The range of what prescriptions are allowed is different between the states. Total ability for prescriptions includes the capability to get a federal DEA registration number.

Nurse practitioner privileges

Depending upon the state's nurse practice act, nurse practitioner (NP) privileges vary:
- NPs may be able to practice independently or in collaboration/agreement with a physician, podiatrist, or chiropractor. The type of physician oversight and collaboration required varies considerably. Only 12 states have no collaboration requirement.
- NPs can be reimbursed by Medicare, Medicaid, The Civilian Health and Medical Program of the Uniformed Services (CHAMPUS), and private insurance. Currently, governmental reimbursement for NPs is at the rate of 85% of the customary physician reimbursement. However, a billing rate of 100% is allowed with "incident to" billing that allows the physician to charge for services that are incident to practice as though he/she performed the service.
- Prescriptive authority varies from state to state. Many states require physician oversight for all or some prescriptions. There are often limits to the types of treatments/drugs that can be prescribed. Only 11 states and Washington, D.C. allow NPs to be completely independent in prescribing medication.

Care process, establishing priorities, and collaboration

The nurse practitioner (NP) is guided by the standards of advance practice, which provide the framework for practice and describes the NP's responsibilities, related to the values and priorities of the profession:
- Care process: In assessing, diagnosing, developing, and implementing a plan of care, as well as evaluating the patient's response, the NP must use scientific method and national standards as the basis for care.
- Establishing priorities: Providing education and encouraging the patient/family to take an active role in self-care is of primary concern. The NP must ensure that the patient can make informed decisions. The NP must assist the patient through all aspects of health care to ensure patient safety and optimal care.
- Collaboration: The NP is a member of the interdisciplinary health team and consults with others when appropriate and refers the patient to specialists as needed. When collaboration is mandated by law, the NP complies with all requirements.

Prescription medication and diagnostic tests

Both prescribing medications and treatment and ordering diagnostic tests are within the scope of practice of nurse practitioners but, as with other aspects of practice, each state establishes how that will be carried out. Additionally, insurance reimbursement varies from 1 area to another and must be considered:

- Prescription: Terminology varies from state to state with nurse practitioners allowed to "furnish" or "prescribe" some types of medications. In some states they may do so independently; in others, they must be "supervised" by a physician under whose auspices they provide care to patients. The nurse practitioner should maintain a list of medications and consider cost-effectiveness when ordering medications.
- Diagnostics: Nurse practitioners can order laboratory, electrocardiogram, and radiographic tests for routine screening and health assessment as well as make a diagnosis based on assessment. There are limitations, depending upon the individual state nursing practice act.

Consultation, referral, and coordination

As part of the scope of practice, the nurse practitioner is able to provide and augment primary care to patients/families through a number of different services:

- Consultation services may include a variety of services, such as assessment of growth, development, and risk factors; providing interventions, (e.g., diet and exercise programs); and educating patients/families.
- Referral services include referring patients to physicians, such as specialists, and to organizations or agencies, such as drug rehabilitation programs.
- Coordination services, with the nurse maintaining contact and receiving reports from referrals in order to provide an integrated plan of care, serves as a valuable service to patients/families, who often must deal with many different healthcare providers who have little or no contact with each other. This type of service can prevent unnecessary duplications of service but also ensure that findings are not overlooked.

Nursing Code of Ethics

The American Nurses Association (ANA) developed the Nursing Code of Ethics. There are 9 provisions:

1. The nurse treats all patients with respect and consideration, regardless of social circumstances or health condition.
2. The nurse's primary commitment is to the patient regardless of conflicts that may arise.
3. The nurse promotes and advocates for the patient's health, safety, and rights, maintaining privacy, confidentiality, and protecting them from questionable practices or care.
4. The nurse is responsible for his/her own care practices and determines appropriate delegation of care.
5. The nurse must retain respect for self and his/her own integrity and competence.
6. The nurse participates in ensuring that the healthcare environment is conducive to providing good health care and consistent with professional and ethical values.
7. The nurse participates in education and knowledge development to advance the profession.
8. The nurse collaborates with others to promote efforts to meet health needs.
9. The nursing profession articulates values and promotes and maintains the integrity of the profession.

Organizations for psychiatric and mental health nurse practitioners

National and international organizations are available for psychiatric and mental health nurse practitioners. Many of these organizations have annual meetings where the newest information on the forefront of mental health nursing is presented. There are membership fees to join these associations:

- The American Psychiatric Nurses Association (APNA) is the largest psychiatric nursing organization. The APNA focuses upon the advancement of nursing practice along with continued improvements in cultural diversity, families, groups, and communities.
- The International Society of Psychiatric-Mental Health Nurses (ISPN) comprises 3 specialty divisions, which include the Association of Child and Adolescent Psychiatric Nurses, the International Society of Psychiatric Consultation Liaison Nurses, and the Society for Education and Research in Psychiatric-Mental Health Nursing. The main goal of the ISPN is to bring together all psychiatric-mental health nurses and to advance quality care available for both the individual and the family unit.

ANA Social Policy Statement

The American Nurses Association (ANA) Social Policy Statement was originally written in 1980, revised in 1995, and again in 2003. The ANA Social Policy Statement provides a description and definition of nursing practice and outlines the knowledge base required for nursing and requirements and scope of practice for advance practice nurses, such as the nurse practitioner. The ANA Social Policy Statement recognizes the social contract that exists between nursing and society and the responsibilities that entails. Nursing requires a holistic approach rather than a problem-focused approach to care, integrating objective data and knowledge and utilizing the scientific method. The ANA Social Policy Statement also describes regulation of nursing, including self-regulation, professional, and legal, centering on the code of ethics, and meeting of certification requirements. Nurses are accountable for their actions under the law but also must assume personal responsibility for maintaining their knowledge base.

Delegation of tasks to unlicensed assistive personnel

The scope of nursing practice includes delegation of tasks to unlicensed assistive personnel, providing those personnel have adequate training and knowledge to carry out the tasks. Delegation should be used to manage the workload and to provide adequate and safe care. The nurse practitioner who delegates remains accountable for patient outcomes and for supervision of the person to whom the task was delegated, so the nurse must consider the following:

- Whether knowledge, skills, and training of the unlicensed assistive personnel provides the ability to perform the delegated task.
- Whether the patient's condition and needs have been properly evaluated and assessed.
- Whether the nurse is able to provide ongoing supervision.

Delegation should be done in a manner that reduces liability by providing adequate communication. This includes specific directions about the task, including what needs to be done, when, and for how long. Expectations related to consultation, reporting, and completion of tasks should be clearly defined. The nurse practitioner should be available to assist if necessary.

Duty to warn

While the law is very clear on issues related to privacy and confidentiality, there are some exceptions related to a duty to warn if the patient poses a danger. Under law, the mental healthcare provider must breach confidentiality if the patient poses a serious risk to him/herself or others. This regulation resulted from a court ruling, Tarasoff v Regents of the University of California (1976), in which the court ruled that the university therapists were negligent when they did not report that a patient was obsessed with Tatiana Tarasoff. When the patient subsequently attacked and killed Tarasoff, her family filed suit against the university and those involved. This issue is somewhat of a gray area, as vague or general statements may not constitute actual threats. The mental healthcare provider must exercise "reasonable" care and report any direct threats to potential victims and indications of suicidal ideation to family/caregivers/authorities.

Least restrictive environment

The Olmstead Decision (1999) by the Supreme Court ensures that disabled patients, including mental health patients, be kept in the least restrictive environment—an integrated environment that allows the patient to interact with those who are not disabled as much as possible and that is appropriate to the needs of the patient. This decision applies to all those protected from discriminatory acts by Title II of the Americans with Disabilities Act (ADA). Under this decision, states must provide community-based services when healthcare professionals deem it appropriate, when the patient agrees, and when placement can be accommodated, considering the resources available. States may be in compliance if they have an effective plan in place for placing patients in the least restrictive environment, but states are allowed a waiting list if the wait is not excessive. Because the decision did not allocate additional funding, resources in some areas are limited.

Autonomy and justice

Autonomy is the ethical principle that the individual has the right to make decisions about his/her own care. In the case of children or mental incompetence, the person cannot make autonomous decisions, so the parents/guardians serve as the legal decision maker. The nurse practitioner must keep patients/parents/guardians fully informed so that they can exercise their autonomy in informed decision making. Justice is the ethical principle that relates to the distribution of the limited resources of healthcare benefits to the members of society. These resources must be distributed fairly. This issue may arise if there is only 1 bed left and 2 sick patients. Justice comes into play in deciding which patient should stay and which should be transported or otherwise cared for. The decision should be made according to what is best or most just for the patients and not colored by personal bias.

Beneficence and nonmaleficence

Beneficence is an ethical principle that involves performing actions that are for the purpose of benefitting another person. In the care of a patient, any procedure or treatment should be done with the ultimate goal of benefitting the patient, and any actions that are not beneficial should be reconsidered. As a patient's condition changes, procedures need to be continually reevaluated to determine if they are still of benefit.

Non-maleficence is an ethical principle that means healthcare workers should provide care in a manner that does not cause direct intentional harm to the patient:

- The actual act must be good or morally neutral.
- The intent must be only for a good effect.
- A bad effect cannot serve as the means to get to a good effect.
- A good effect must have more benefit than a bad effect has harm.

Boundaries

When the boundary between the role of the nurse practitioner and the vulnerability of the patient is breached, a boundary violation occurs. Because the nurse practitioner is in the position of "authority," the responsibility to maintain the boundary rests with the nurse; however, the line separating them is a continuum and sometimes not easily defined.

Sexual
It is inappropriate for nurse practitioners to engage in sexual relations with patients, and if the sexual behavior is coerced or the patient cognitively impaired, it is illegal. However, more common violations with older adults or mentally incompetent adults include exposing a patient unnecessarily, using sexually demeaning gestures or language (including off-color jokes), harassment, or inappropriate touching. Touching should be used with care, such as touching a hand or shoulder. Hugging may be misconstrued.

Gifts
Over time, patients may develop a bond with nurse practitioners they trust and may feel grateful to the nurse practitioner for the care provided and want to express thanks, but the nurse practitioner must make sure to maintain professional boundaries. Patients often offer gifts to nurse practitioners to show their appreciation, but older adults, especially those who are weak and ill or have cognitive impairment, may be taken advantage of easily. Patients may offer valuables and may sometimes be easily manipulated into giving large sums of money. Small tokens of appreciation that can be shared with other staff, such as a box of chocolates, are usually acceptable (depending upon the policy of the institution), but almost any other gifts (jewelry, money, clothes) should be declined: "I'm sorry, that's so kind of you, but nurses are not allowed to accept gifts from patients." Declining may relieve the patient of the feeling of obligation.

Attention
Nursing is a giving profession, but the nurse practitioner must temper giving with recognition of professional boundaries. Patients have many needs; and, as acts of kindness, nurse practitioners, especially those involved in home care, often give them extra attention, may offer to do favors such as cooking or shopping, and may become overly invested in the patients' lives. While this may benefit a patient in the short term, it can establish a relationship of increasing dependency and obligation that does not resolve the long-term needs of the patient. Making referrals to the appropriate agencies or collaborating with family to find ways to provide services is more effective. Becoming overly invested may be evident by the nurse showing favoritism or spending too much time with the patient while neglecting other duties. On the other end of the spectrum are nurse practitioners who are disinterested and fail to provide adequate attention to the patient's detriment. Lack of adequate attention may lead to outright neglect.

Coercion

Power issues are inherent in matters associated with professional boundaries. Physical abuse is both unprofessional and illegal, but behavior can easily border on abusive without the patient being physically injured. Nurse practitioners can easily intimidate patients into having procedures or treatments they don't want. Regardless of age, patients have the right to choose and the right to refuse treatment. Difficulties arise with cognitive impairment, and in that case, another responsible adult (often a child, parent, or spouse) is designated to make decisions, but every effort should be made to gain patient cooperation. Forcing the patient to do something against his/her will borders on abuse and can sometimes degenerate into actual abuse if physical coercion is involved.

Personal information

When pre-existing personal or business relationships exist, other nurse practitioners should be assigned care of the patient whenever possible, but this may be difficult in small communities. However, the practitioner should strive to maintain a professional role separate from the personal role and respect professional boundaries:
- Personal information: The nurse practitioner must respect and maintain the confidentiality of the patient and family members, but must also be very careful about disclosing personal information about himself/herself because this establishes a social relationship that interferes with the professional role of the nurse and the boundary between the patient and the nurse. The nurse practitioner and patient should never share "secrets." When the nurse practitioner divulges personal information, he/she may become vulnerable to the patient, resulting in a reversal of roles.

Advance directives, DNR, and durable power of attorney

In accordance to Federal and state laws, individuals have the right to self-determination in health care, including decisions about end-of-life care through advance directives such as living wills and the right to assign a surrogate person to make decisions through a durable power of attorney. Patients should routinely be questioned about an advanced directive as they may present at a healthcare organization without the document. Patients who have indicated they desire a do-not-resuscitate (DNR) order should not receive resuscitative treatments for terminal illness or conditions in which meaningful recovery cannot occur. Patients and families of those with terminal illnesses should be questioned as to whether the patients are Hospice patients. For those with DNR requests or those withdrawing life support, staff should provide the patient palliative rather than curative measures, such as pain control and/or oxygen, and emotional support to the patient and family. Religious traditions and beliefs about death should be treated with respect.

Privacy

The Health Insurance Portability and Accountability Act (HIPAA) addresses the rights of the individual related to privacy of health information. The nurse practitioner must not release any information or documentation about a patient's condition or treatment without consent, as the individual has the right to determine who has access to personal information. Personal information about the patient is considered protected health information (PHI), and consists of any identifying or personal information about the patient, such as health history, condition, or treatments in any form and any documentation, including electronic, verbal, or written. Personal information can be shared with spouse, legal guardians, those with durable power of attorney for the patient, and those involved in care of the patient (ie, physicians) without a specific release, but the patient should always be consulted if personal information is to be discussed with others present to ensure there is no objection. Failure to comply with HIPAA regulations can make a nurse practitioner liable for legal action.

ADA

The 1992 Americans with Disabilities Act (ADA) is civil rights legislation that provides the disabled, including those with mental impairment, access to employment and the community. While employers must make reasonable accommodations for the disabled, the provisions related to the community apply more directly to older Americans. The ADA covers not only obvious disabilities but also disorders such as arthritis, seizure disorders, psychiatric disorders, cardiovascular, and respiratory disorders. Communities must provide transportation services for the disabled, including accommodation for wheelchairs. Public facilities (schools, museums, physician's offices, post offices, restaurants) must be accessible with ramps and elevators as needed. Telecommunications must also be accessible through devices or accommodations for the deaf and blind. Compliance is not yet complete because older buildings are required to provide access that is possible without "undue hardship," but newer construction of public facilities must meet ADA regulations.

Patient Self-Determination Act

The Patient Self-Determination Act (1990), an amendment to the Omnibus Budget Reconciliation Act, allows a mental health patient to develop an advance psychiatric directive (APD) during a period when a professional mental healthcare provider certifies the person is of sound mind. The APD allows the patient to determine in advance the types of treatment that are acceptable and those that are not. The patient can also designate another person, such as a family member, to make decisions if the patient is unable to do so. State regulations regarding APDs may vary somewhat. The APD is particularly valuable to those who have severe chronic psychiatric illnesses, such as schizophrenia, and may face involuntary commitment. A patient may outline preferences regarding specific treatments and interventions, such as medications, seclusion, restraint, and electroshock therapy.

Informed consent

Patients or family must provide informed consent for all treatment the patient receives. This consent includes a thorough explanation of all procedures and treatment and associated risks. Patients/family should be apprised of all options and allowed input on the type of treatments. Patients/family should be apprised of all reasonable risks and any complications that might be life threatening or increase morbidity. The American Medical Association has established guidelines for informed consent:
- Explanation of diagnosis.
- Nature and reason for treatment or procedure.
- Risks and benefits.
- Alternative options (regardless of cost or insurance coverage).
- Risks and benefits of alternative options.
- Risks and benefits of not having a treatment or procedure.
- Providing informed consent is a requirement of all states.

Risk management

Risk management is an organized and formal method of decreasing liability, financial loss, and risk or harm to patients, staff, or others by doing an assessment of risk and introducing risk-management strategies. Much of risk management has been driven by the insurance industry in order to minimize costs, but quality management utilizes risk management as a method to ensure quality health care and process improvement. An organization's risk management program usually comprises a manager and staff with a number of responsibilities:

- Risk identification begins with an assessment of processes to identify and prioritize those that require further study to determine risk exposure.
- Risk analysis requires a careful documenting of process and utilizing flow charts, with each step in the process assessed for potential risks. This may utilize root cause analysis methods.
- Risk prevention involves instituting corrective or preventive processes. Responsible individual or teams are identified and trained.
- Assessment/evaluation of corrective/preventive processes is ongoing to determine if they are effective or require modification.

Malpractice

Nurse practitioners (NPs), as all advance practice nurses, are usually insured for malpractice at a higher rate than for registered nurses because their scope of practice is much wider. An NP may be sued individually or as part of a medical group to which the NP is associated. Because a suit is a civil matter, loss of judgment may not be reported to the state board of nursing. If a charge of negligence is brought to the attention of the board, the board may initiate an investigation and disciplinary action. Negligence may involve a number of failures, such as not referring a patient when needed, incorrect diagnosis, incorrect treatment, and not providing the patient/family with adequate or essential information. Once a NP has established a duty to a patient—by direct examination or even casual or telephone conversation that involves professional advice—the NP may be liable for malpractice if he/she doe not follow-up with adequate care.

Chally and Loriz model for ethical decision making

It is important for nurse practitioners to avoid making decisions solely based on their beliefs that they know what is best for patients. In 1998, Chally and Loriz developed a model for ethical decision making for nurse practitioners to use when faced with ethical dilemmas or choices. Steps to ethical decision making include:

1. Clarifying the extent/type of dilemma and who is ultimately responsible for making the decision.
2. Obtaining more data, including information about legal issues, such as the obligation to report.
3. Considering alternative solutions.
4. Arriving at a decision after considering risk/benefits and discussing it with the patient.
5. Acting on the decision and utilizing collaboration as needed.
6. Assessing the outcomes of the decision to determine if the chosen action was effective.

Ethical dilemmas

While the terms ethics and morals are sometimes used interchangeably, ethics is a study of morals and encompasses concepts of right and wrong. When dealing with ethical dilemmas, one must consider not only what people should do but also what they actually do, as these 2 things are sometimes at odds. Ethical issues can be difficult to assess because of personal bias, and that is 1 of the reasons that sharing concerns with other internal sources and reaching consensus is so valuable. Issues of concern might include options for care, refusal of care, rights to privacy, adequate relief of suffering, and the right to self-determination. Internal sources might include the ethics committee, whose charge is to make decisions regarding ethical issues. Risk management can provide guidance related to personal and institutional liability. External agencies might include government agencies, such as the public health department.

Environment for ethical decision-making and patient advocacy

An environment for ethical decision-making and patient advocacy does not appear when it is needed; it requires planning and preparation. The expectation for the institution should clearly communicate that nurses are legally and morally responsible for assuring competent care and respecting the rights of patients and other stakeholders. Decisions regarding ethical issues often must be made quickly with little time for contemplation; therefore, ethical issues that may arise should be identified and discussed. Clearly defined procedures and policies for dealing with conflicts, including an active ethics committee, in-service training, and staff meetings, must be established. Patients and families need to be part of the ethical environment, which means empowering them by providing patient/family information (e.g., print form, video, audio) that outlines patient's rights and procedures for expressing their wishes and dealing with ethical conflicts. Respect for privacy and confidentiality and a nonpunitive atmosphere are essential.

Resolving ethical conflicts

In the health care setting, it is important that ethical conflicts be resolved without harming the patient or compromising care. There are several factors that will affect the course and outcome of an ethical conflict. First, the level of commitment the clinician has to the patient will determine the amount of effort put forth in resolving an ethical conflict. Second, the degree of moral certainty the clinician has will determine the approach to resolution; if the clinician feels that he or she is correct, he or she will most likely not waver in the decision. Third, the amount of time available for resolution is important; if the clinician is pressed for time, he or she will most likely come to a decision faster than if there is not a time constraint, in which case avoidance may occur. Fourth is the cost-benefit ratio; if the patient refuses to negotiate a certain point, for example, it is not worth the time to the clinician to try to influence the patient's decision.

Ethical issues of competency and decision-making

Competence and incompetence are legal issues, not diagnostic. In order to give informed consent, a patient is supposed to be competent enough to understand the issues to which the person is consenting. However, some psychiatric patients are not competent enough to make decisions about treatment; but, unless a person is a minor, is unable to respond, or has been declared legally incompetent, the ethical principle of autonomy applies, meaning that the person has the right to make decisions about treatment and care—even if those decisions are not in the person's best interests. In most states, involuntary commitment, which occurs without patient consent, is only allowed in emergency situations in which the person poses a threat to self or others, for observation and treatment (as decreed by the courts), and when a patient is so gravely disabled that the person cannot take care of personal needs. Emergency commitments are usually only for 72 hours, at which time the patient must have a competency hearing.

Ethical issue of unavailable resources

The issue of unavailable resources as it applies to psychiatric care relates to the ethical principal of justice, which deals with the distribution of limited healthcare resources. According to this principle, distribution should be based on decisions that are the most just and should not reflect personal bias, attempting to make objective decisions when decision-making is inherently subjective. All individuals in need of psychiatric care should have equal access, and if resources are limited, those in greatest need should be provided healthcare services first. However, the reality is that there is little equal access. People with insurance or the means to pay privately are often treated first and usually have access to the best care. People without the means to pay often have little access to care, a long wait for care, or substandard care. Psychiatric care for the uninsured often takes place in over-crowded and understaffed facilities.

Human subject protection

The Food and Drug Administration, Code of Federal Regulations, Title 21, Volume 1, regulates protection of human subjects and states that any researcher involving patients in research must obtain informed consent, in language understandable to the patient or the patient's agent. The elements of this informed consent must include an explanation of the research, the purpose, and the expected duration, as well as a description off any potential risks. Potential benefits must be described and possible alternative treatments. Any compensation to be provided must be outlined. The extent of confidentiality should be clarified. Contact information should be provided in the event the patient/family has questions. The patient must be informed that participation is voluntary and that he/she can discontinue participation at any time without penalty. Informed consent must be documented by a signed, written agreement.

Peck's theory of adult development

Peck expanded on Erikson's stages of adult development, believing that there were 7 important tasks that were required during the last 2 stages of life:

Stage	Tasks	Outcomes
Middle age	Valuing wisdom vs physical powers. Socializing vs sex-ualizing. Cathectic (libidinal energy) flexibility vs cathectic impover-ishment. Mental flexibility vs mental rigidity.	*Negative* outcomes lead to weak relationships, inflexibility, and resistance to change. *Positive* outcomes lead to strong relationships, flexibility in lifestyle, and adaptability to change.
Older adult-hood	Ego differentiation vs work role preoccupation. Body transcen-dence vs body preoccupation. Ego transcendence vs ego preoccupation.	*Negative* outcomes leads to feel-ing of loss of identity after retiring, depression, inability to accept bodily/functional changes and fear of death. *Positive* outcomes lead to meaningful life after retirement, acceptance of bodily/functional changes, acceptance of death, and feeling that life has been good.

Erikson's Theory of Psychological Development

Erikson's Theory of Psychosocial Development covers the life span, focusing on conflicts at each stage and the virtue that is the outcome of finding a balance in the conflict. The first 5 stages relate to infancy and childhood and the last 3 stages to adulthood, but childhood development affects later adult development:

Trust vs mistrust	Birth to 1 year	Can result in mistrust or faith and optimism.
Autonomy vs shame/doubt	1-3 years	Can lead to doubt and shame or self-control and willpower.
Initiative vs guilt	3-6 years	Can lead to guilt or direction and purpose.
Industry vs inferiority	6-12 years	Can lead to inadequacy and inferiority or competence.
Identify vs role confusion	12-18 years	Can lead to role confusion or devotion and fidelity to others.
Intimacy vs isolation	Young adulthood	Can lead to lack of close relationships or love/intimacy.
Generativity vs stagnation	Middle age	Can lead to stagnation or caring and achievements.
Ego integrity vs despair	Older adulthood	Can lead to despair (failure to accept changes of aging) or wisdom (acceptance).

Continuity theory and life-course theory

Continuity
Havighurst, Neugarten, and Tobin believed that neither activity theory nor disengagement theory was adequate from a sociological perspective to explain successful aging and that personality type correlated with adjustment to aging. People maintain continuity in their adaptation to changing roles according to their basic personality type:
- Integrated: Individuals adjust well to aging and changing roles and remain active.
- Armored-defended: Individuals maintain roles and activities they had during middle age and with which they feel secure.
- Passive-dependent: Individuals become increasingly dependent on others and/or are passive in their changing roles.
- Unintegrated: Individuals are unable to cope well with aging.

Life course
This theory contends that aging is a lifelong process of social, psychological, and biological changes that begin with infancy and continue through older adulthood, viewed within cultural, economic, social, and historic context.

Resiliency Theory

The Resiliency Theory describes the ability of children to function in healthy ways despite adverse circumstances. This theory explains the dynamics of response to a crisis, considering the characteristics inherent in the individual as well as the environmental characteristics. When a crisis occurs, the child (along with his or her family) encounters vulnerability, stress, and increased risks in coping. Families respond in different manners, sometimes relying on extended family or coping with abnormal behavior (such as an alcoholic parent). Children and families also have protective factors (such as faith, previous experience, supportive family members, etc) that provide assistance in coping with changes. The family often goes through a phase of adjustment to changes, during which they may be disorganized and unable to cope, but this evolves to an adaptation phase during which the child and family appraise the situation and use problem solving to arise at a positive or negative response to the change.

Maslow's hierarchy of needs and Jung's theory of individualism

Hierarchy of needs
Maslow stated that human behavior is motivated by needs and that there is a hierarchy of needs that begin with basic needs and progress to personal needs. The hierarchy includes:
- Physiological needs (the base)
- Safety and security
- Belonging
- Self-esteem
- Self-actualization (the apex)

People may not progress in 1 direction from 1 need to another but movement may be in multiple directions in a lifelong process of working toward self-actualization, which requires creativity and some degree of freedom. Failure to develop toward self-actualization may result in depression and feelings of failure.

Theory of individualism
Jung theorized that personality developed over the lifespan. Personality comprises ego, personal unconsciousness, and collective unconsciousness. Personality can be introverted or extroverted, but a balance is necessary for emotional health. Jung theorized that during middle age, people begin to question their values, beliefs, and attainments. As they continue to age, they turn more inward. Successful aging is when people value themselves more than the concern they have for external things, losses, and physical limitations.

Problems during school-age years

During the years of 6-12, routine health assessments should be done at ages 6, 8, 10, 11, and 12 to determine if there are developmental delays or problems, which may include:
- 6 years: Peer problems, depression, cruelty to animals, poor academic progress, speech problems, lack of fine motor skills, and inability to catch a ball or state age.
- 8 years: No close friends, depression, cruelty to animals, interest in fires, very poor academic progress with inability to do math, read or write adequately, and poor coordination.
- 10 years: No team sports and poor choices in peers (gangs), failure to follow rules, cruelty to animals and interest in fires, depression, failure to understand causal relationships, poor academic progress in reading, writing, math, penmanship, and problems throwing or catching.
- 11-12 years: Continuation of problems at 10 years with increasing risk-taking behaviors (drinking, drugs, sex) and continued poor academic progress in reading, following directions, doing homework, and organization.

Issues for early adolescence

Early adolescence, 11-14, is a transitional time for children as their hormones and bodies go through changes. Children mature at varying rates, so there are wide differences. Emotions may be labile, and the child may feel isolated and confused at times, trying to find an identity. Peers take on more influence and the child may challenge the values of the family. Children may have much anxiety about their bodies and sexuality as secondary sexual characteristics develops. Developmental concerns include:
- Delayed maturation.
- Short stature (females).
- Spinal curvature (females).
- Poor dental status (caries, malocclusion).
- Chronic illnesses, such as diabetes.
- Lack of adequate physical activity.
- Poor nutrition, anorexia.
- Concerns about sexual identity.
- Negative self-image.
- Depression.
- Lack of close friends, fighting, or violent episodes.
- Poor academic progress with truancy and failure to complete assignments.
- Lack of impulse control.

Issues for middle adolescence

In middle adolescence, ages 15-17, most body changes have occurred, and there is less concern about this but more concern about the image they are projecting to others. Girls may worry about weight and boys about muscle development. Teenagers are interested in sexuality and many begin sexual experimentation. There is strong identification with peer groups, including codes of dress and behavior, often putting them at odds with family. Developmental concerns include:
- Spinal curvature (females) and short stature (males).
- Lack of testicular maturation/persistent gynecomastia.
- Acne.
- Anorexia, obesity.
- Sexual experimentation, multiple partners, and unprotected sex.
- Sexual identification concerns.
- Depression, poor self-image.
- Lack of adequate exercise, poor nutrition, and poor dental health.
- Chronic diseases.
- Experimentation with drugs and alcohol and problems with authority figures.
- Lack of peer group identification, gang association.
- Poor academic progress, failing classes, truancy, attention deficits and disruptive class behavior, poor judgment, and impulse control.

Issues for late adolescence

Late adolescence, 18-21, is the time when adolescents begin to take on more adult roles and responsibilities, entering the world of work or going to college. Most have come to terms with their sexuality and have a more mature understanding of people's motivations. Some young people will continue to engage in high-risk behaviors. Many of the problems associated with middle

adolescence may continue if unresolved, interfering with the transition to adulthood. Developmental concerns include:
- Failure to take on adult roles, no life goals or future plans.
- Low self-esteem.
- Lack of intimate relationships, sexual identification concerns.
- Gang association.
- Continued identification with peer group or dependence on parents.
- High-risk sexual behavior, multiple partners, and unprotected sex.
- Poor academic progress or ability.
- Psychosomatic complaints, depression.
- Lack of impulse control.
- Poor nutrition, obesity, anorexia.
- Poor dental health.
- Chronic disease.
- Lack of exercise.

Cognitive changes associated with normal aging

Cognitive changes related to age vary among individuals but are usually not evident until >70. Studies have shown that by age 81, about 60-70% of people have a small decline in cognitive abilities. Fluid intelligence (information processing skills) tends to decline slightly with age while crystallized intelligence (acquired knowledge and applied problem solving) is more likely to stay intact and may even improve. Older adults may have more difficulty in completing complex tasks that require processing of new information. They may become more easily distracted and less able to focus attention. Processing information and reacting may be slowed so that those >60 require more time to complete mental tasks even though their intellectual capability remains intact. Working memory declines making it more difficult for older adults to complete mental processes that require keeping facts in memory (such as calculating costs and tips). Implicit memories (skills, reactions) usually remain intact while explicit memories (facts, information) may decline. Older adults often have difficulty retrieving words (names of people or objects).

Neuroprotective strategies

Neuroprotective strategies are those used to prevent damage to the brain. Strategies include:
- Substance abuse programs: Dual diagnosis is common, but substance abuse may worsen symptoms and interfere with recovery or maintenance, so patients should be referred to substance abuse programs specifically intended for those with mental illness.
- Medication choice: Atypical antipsychotics are less likely to result in extrapyramidal adverse effects than typical but more likely to result in metabolic effects and weight gain, which may lead to cardiovascular disease and diabetes. Patients should be maintained on drugs for psychotic episodes at least one year and many may need drugs indefinitely. Patients must learn to recognize signs of relapse. Restarting medications immediately on relapse can prevent symptoms from becoming severe.
- Cognitive behavioral therapy: Can help patients learn to control symptoms and recognize hallucinations and delusions, allowing them to function better in society.
- Early intervention: The prognosis for mental disorders is better if treatment is instituted early, with the first episode, rather than delayed.
- Support programs: Programs to support patients in the community increase compliance with treatment.

Risk assessment

A risk assessment evaluates the patient's condition and situation for the presence of certain risk factors. These risks can be influenced by age, ethnicity, spiritual or social beliefs and can include risk for suicide, harming others, exacerbation of symptoms, development of new mental health issues, falls, seizures, or allergic reactions. This assessment should occur within the first hour of their arrival and then continue as an ongoing process. The patient's specific risks should be prioritized, documented, and then nursing interventions should be put into place to protect the patient or others. Two of the most important areas to evaluate are the patient's risk for self harm or harm to others. The staff member performing the assessment should very closely evaluate for any descriptions or thoughts the patient may have concerning these risks. Direct questioning on these subjects should be performed and documented. If the patient admits having these thoughts or ideas, the patient must be placed in close monitoring for either suicidal or assaultive precautions per facility protocol.

Risk factors

Malnutrition
There are a number of risk factors for malnutrition:
- Hypermetabolism resulting from various diseases, such as acquired immune deficiency syndrome (AIDS), and trauma, stress, or infection.
- Weight loss, especially sudden or loss of 10% of normal weight over a 3-month period.
- Low body weight, defined as <90% of ideal body weight for age.
- Low Body Mass Index (BMI), defined as <18.5.
- Immunosuppressive drugs, which interfere with absorption of nutrients.
- Malabsorption of nutrients caused by diseases, such as chronic failure of kidneys or liver.
- Changes in appetite that decrease intake of nutrients.
- Food intolerances, such as lactose intolerance, resulting from lack of enzymes needed to completely digest food so it can be absorbed into the blood stream from the small intestine.
- Dietary restrictions, such as limited intake of protein with kidney failure.
- Functional limitations, such as inability to feed oneself.
- Lack of teeth or dentures, limiting intake.
- Alterations of taste or smell that render food unpalatable.

Tardive dyskinesia
Tardive dyskinesia (TD) is caused by typical antipsychotics and affects overall about 20% of patients receiving these drugs; however, older adults (>50) are more severely impacted with rates of 50 to 70% in those receiving antipsychotic drugs. Females are more likely to suffer TD than males. Other risk factors include:
- Depression and other affective disorders.
- Brain injury.
- Pro-longed treatment and/or excessively high doses (prevalence increases about 5% per year of treatment).
- Standard antipsychotics (such as haloperidol).

Symptoms usually begin after 6 months of treatment or withdrawal of medication and include abnormal movements, such as lip smacking and blinking, muscle twitching, hair pulling, and protruding tongue. Symptoms are often irreversible but if associated with reduction or withdrawal of medication, usually resolve within 3 months.

Falling

There are both physical and psychological deficits or abnormalities that can contribute to a patient's fall risk. Physical factors include weakness, lower extremity abnormalities that could negatively affect gait or ability to bear weight, diarrhea or urinary urgency or frequency, or altered mental status due to medications, electrolyte imbalances, infection, or hypoxia. Psychological alterations that can increase the patient's fall risk can include dementia, delirium, other confusional states, paranoia, or suicidal ideations. Environmental factors can also increase risk for a fall. These factors may include: lack of adequate lighting, lack of adequate footwear, bed raised to a high position, unfamiliar environment, call bell not within easy reach, or use of restraints. All of these factors should be evaluated to provide the safest environment possible to prevent patient injury.

Emotional and mental disorders in children and adolescents

Psychiatric illness occurs in about 10% of children before age 18; although only about 20% receive treatment. Risk factors for emotional and mental disorders in children and adolescents include:

- Exposure to environmental toxins, such as high levels of lead.
- Living in poverty or crowded inner-city locations.
- Exposure to violence, such as witnessing or being the victim of physical or sexual abuse, drive-by shootings, muggings, etc.
- A child of a parent who is a substance abuser or who is mentally ill.
- Children of a teenage parent.
- Children with a chronic disease or a disability.
- Children exposed to prolonged separation from parent(s).
- Children with multiple separations from parent(s).
- Children who experience frequent changes in primary caretakers.
- Homelessness.
- Children who experience the loss of significant others through death, divorce, or broken relationships.

Anger, aggression, and violence

Psychological aspects of increased anger, aggression, and violence can be associated with uncontrollable instinctual urges or as a result of the person's particular life experiences. Exposure to violence, altered mother/child bonding, altered socialization skills, or reinforcement of aggressive behavior by achievement of a goal can all lead to increased utilization of aggression and violence. Over exposure to violence through the media, entertainment, or the immediate environment can possibly lead to a desensitization of aggression and violence and lead to maladaptive behavioral responses. During an assessment, the background history of a patient can reveal many different predictors of future maladaptive responses associated with aggression and violence. The history may reveal violent behaviors and rage responses, increasing irritability, or loss of control. Some examples of maladaptive background behaviors include: cruelty to animals or children, setting fires or other destruction of property, drug or alcohol abuse, self directed violence, such as cuts or burns on the arms, or juvenile delinquency. Many of these behaviors are evident during childhood.

Acute and chronic pain

Pain affects both the physical and psychological well being of the individual. It encompasses both a sensory and emotional response. A patient will cope with pain through many different behavioral responses. Acute pain is associated with an immediate occurring problem and is usually resolved in a few months or less. Fear, expectations, coping abilities, or cultural influences can all affect a patient's response to pain. A change in normal sleep patterns, anorexia, anxiety, or agitation can occur. Chronic pain is pain that lasts longer than 6 months. Chronic pain can lead to neurochemical abnormalities and depression. A complete assessment and evaluation of the pain should be performed and documented. Appropriate diagnosis and treatment plan should be in place to assist with successful treatment of pain.

<u>Biological risk factors for mental illness</u>
Biological factors affect one's predisposition for mental illness. In addition to genetics, maternal and fetal health during pregnancy and exposure to environmental toxins before the age of 6 can affect mental health. Peripartum concerns, including poor nutrition, maternal stress, drug use, and poor living conditions may contribute to biological risk for mental illness. Mental and physical retardation, developmental deficits, and deformities may also increase the risk for mental illness. Tumors, trauma, and degenerative processes of the brain may cause structural or chemical changes within the brain that result in mental disorders. Biological factors can interact with other influences, such as a family history of violence, drug or alcohol abuse, schizophrenia, or non-compliance with medication regimens.

Neglect and lack of supervised care in children

While some children may not be physically or sexually abused, they may suffer from profound neglect or lack of supervision that places them at risk. Indicators include:
- Appearing dirty and unkempt, sometimes with infestations of lice, and wearing ill fitting, torn clothing and shoes.
- Being tired and sleepy during the daytime.
- Having excessive medical or dental problems, such as extensive dental caries.
- Missing appointments and not receiving proper immunizations.
- Being underweight for their current stage of development.

Neglect can be difficult to assess, especially if the nurse practitioner is serving a homeless or very disadvantaged population. Home visits may be needed to ascertain if there is adequate food, clothing, or supervision, and this may be beyond the scope of care provided by the nurse practitioner. Thus, suspicions should be reported so that a follow-up assessment of the home environment can be done.

Physical and behavioral signs of physical abuse in children

Children rarely admit to being abused and, in fact, typically deny it and attempt to protect the abusing parent. Therefore, the nurse practitioner must often rely on physical and behavioral signs to determine if there is cause to suspect physical abuse:
- Behavioral indicators: The child may be overly compliant or fearful with obvious changes in demeanor when a parent/caregiver is present. Some children act out with aggression toward other children or animals. Children may become depressed, suicidal, or present with sleeping or eating disorders. Behaviors may become increasingly self-destructive as the child ages.

- Physical indicators: The type, location, and extent of injuries can raise suspicion of abuse. Head and facial injuries and bruising are common, as are bite or burn marks. There may be hand prints or grab marks, unusual bruising, such as across the buttocks. Any bruising, swelling, or tearing of the genital area and the identification of sexually transmitted diseases are also causes for concern.

Rape and sexual abuse

Rape and sexual abuse victims (both male and female) should be treated sensitively and questioned privately. Examination should include:
- Assault history that includes what happened, when, where, and by whom. Questioning should determine if there is a possibility of drug-induced amnesia or activities, such as douching or showering, which might have destroyed evidence.
- Medical history to determine if there is a risk of pregnancy and when and if the last consensual sex occurred that might interfere with laboratory findings.
- Physical examination should include examination of the genitals, rectum, and mouth. The body should be examined for bruising or other injuries. Toluidine dye should be applied to the perineum before insertion of a speculum into the vagina to detect small vulvar lacerations.

Forensic evidence must be collected within 72 hours and requires informed consent and the use of a rape kit. Forensic evidence includes:
- Victim samples for control.
- Assailant-identifying samples.
- Evidence of sexual activity.
- Evidence of force or coercion.

Injuries consistent with domestic violence

There are a number of characteristic injuries indicating domestic violence:
- Ruptured eardrum.
- Rectal/genital injury—burns, bites, trauma.
- Scrapes and bruises about the neck, face, head, trunk, arms.
- Cuts, bruises, and fractures of the face.

The pattern of injuries is also often distinctive:
- Bathing suit pattern—injuries on parts of body that are usually covered with clothing as the perpetrator abuses but hides evidence of abuse.
- Head and neck injuries (50%).

Abusive injuries (rarely attributable to accidents) are common:
- Bites, bruises, rope and cigarette burns, welts in the outline of weapons (belt marks).
- Bilateral injuries of arms/legs.

Defensive injuries are indicative of abuse:
- Back of the body injury from being attacked while crouched on the floor face down.
- Soles of the feet from kicking at perpetrator.
- Ulnar aspect of hand or palm from blocking blows.

Domestic violence

According to guidelines of the Family Violence Prevention Fund, assessment for domestic violence should be done for all adolescent and adult patients, regardless of background or signs of abuse. While females are the most common victims, there are increasing reports of male victims of domestic violence, both in heterosexual and homosexual relationships. The person doing the assessment should be informed about domestic violence and be aware of risk factors and danger signs. The interview should be conducted in private (or with children <3 years old). The nurse practitioner's office, bathrooms, and examining rooms should have information about domestic violence posted prominently. Brochures and information should be available to give to patients. Patients may present with a variety of physical complaints, such as headache, pain, palpitations, numbness, or pelvic pain. They are often depressed and may appear suicidal and may be isolated from friends and family. Victims of domestic violence often exhibit fear of spouse/partner and may report injury inconsistent with symptoms.

Family Violence Prevention Fund steps to identifying victims of domestic violence

The Family Violence Prevention Fund has issued guidelines for identifying victims of domestic violence. There are 7 steps:
1. Inquiry: Non-judgmental questioning should begin with asking if the person has ever been abused—physically, sexually, or psychologically.
2. Interview: The person may exhibit signs of anxiety or fear and may blame himself/herself or report that others believe he/she is abused. The person should be questioned if he/she is afraid for his/her life or for children.
3. Question: If the person reports abuse, it is critical to ask if the person is in immediate danger or if the abuser is on the premises. The interviewer should ask if the person has been threatened. The history and pattern of abuse should be questioned, and if children are involved, whether the children are abused. Note: State laws vary, and in some states, it is mandatory to report if a child was present during an act of domestic violence as this is considered child abuse. The nurse practitioner must be aware of state laws regarding domestic and child abuse, and all nurses are mandatory reporters.
4. Validate: The interviewer should offer support and reassurance in a non-judgmental manner, telling the patient the abuse is not his/her fault.
5. Give information: While discussing facts about domestic violence and the tendency to escalate, the interviewer should provide brochures and information about safety planning. If the patient wants to file a complaint with the police, the interviewer should assist the person to place the call.
6. Make referrals: Information about state, local, and national organizations should be provided along with telephone numbers and contact numbers for domestic violence shelters.
7. Document: Record keeping should be legal, legible, and lengthy with complete report and description of any traumatic injuries resulting from domestic violence. A body map may be used to indicate sites of injury, especially if there are multiple bruises or injuries.

Elder abuse

There are many different types of elder abuse: physical (such as hitting or improperly restraining), sexual, psychological, financial, and neglect. Elder abuse may be difficult to diagnose, especially if the person is cognitively impaired, but symptoms can include: fearfulness, disparities in reports of injuries between patient and caregiver, evidence of old or repeated injuries, poor hygiene and dental care, decubiti, malnutrition, undue concern with costs on caregiver's part, unsupportive attitude of caregiver, and caregiver's reluctance or refusal to allow patient to communicate privately with the nurse practitioner. Self-abuse can also occur when patients are not able to adequately care for themselves. Diagnosis of elder abuse includes a careful history and physical exam, including directly questioning the patient about abuse. Treatment includes attending to injuries or physical needs, and this can vary widely, and referral to adult protective services as indicated. Reporting laws regarding elder abuse vary somewhat from one state to another, but all states have laws regarding elder abuse and 42 require mandatory reporting by heath workers.

Suicide risk assessment

A suicide risk assessment should be completed and documented upon admission, with each shift change, at discharge, or any time suicidal ideation is suggested by the patient. This risk assessment should evaluate some of the following criteria: Would the patient sign a contract for safety? Is there a suicide plan? How lethal is the plan? What is the elopement risk? How often are the suicidal thoughts, and has the person attempted suicide before? Any associated symptoms of hopelessness, guilt, anger, helplessness, impulsive behaviors, nightmares, obsession with death, or altered judgment should also be assessed and documented. The higher the score is, the higher the risk for suicide. Patients who actually attempt suicide should be hospitalized and assessed for suicide risk after initial treatment. High-risk findings include:
- Violent suicide attempt (knives, gunshots).
- Suicide attempt with low chance of rescue.
- Ongoing psychosis or disordered thinking.
- Ongoing severe depression and feeling of helplessness.
- History of previous suicide attempts.
- Lack of social support system.

Alcohol use

All patients should be assessed for alcohol use as part of the initial history and physical exam as well as at subsequent visits, especially if there are health indications (abnormal liver function tests, falls, insomnia) or social indications (family problems, divorce, job loss). There are numerous self-assessment screening tools that ask the patient a number of questions about the frequency and amount of drinking as well as questions such as if he/she drinks in the morning or alone; has been arrested, has lost a job, or missed work because of drinking; feels depressed; or if he/she drinks to gain confidence. The assessment tools have a scale indicator that suggests a problem with certain scores. The nurse practitioner should discuss the assessment and score with the patient and provide information about resources (such as Alcoholics Anonymous and alcohol rehabilitation programs) and health consequences of drinking to the patient.

Children and adolescents
Alcohol is a significant problem in adolescence and even in younger children. It is the most-commonly abused substance. Studies have shown that about 32% of young people drink and 20% are binge drinkers. While alcohol can impair development of almost all body systems in a growing child, it is of particular concern for the effects on the neurological system and liver. Additionally, because it interferes with impulse control, adolescents who drink are often involved in violence, abuse, and at-risk sexual behavior. Drinking should be suspected if a child has memory problems, changes in behavior, poor academic progress, emotional lability, and physical changes, such as slurring of speech, general lethargy, or lack of coordination. Intervention includes teaching children

from about age 9 about the dangers of drinking, identifying those who are drinking, identifying underlying problems, and providing programs to help teenagers stop drinking, such as counselling or Alcoholics Anonymous.

Drug use in children and adolescents

Drug use continues to be a serious problem for children and teenagers, with some starting as young as 9 or 10, using a wide variety of drugs, including marijuana, crack, prescription drugs, cocaine, inhalants (such as glue and lighter fluid), hallucinogens, and steroids. Risk factors include aggressive behavior, poor social skills, and poor academic progress coupled with lack of parental supervision, poverty, and availability of drugs. Small children are often reacting to circumstances within the family while teenagers are responding to peer pressure from outside the family. Studies have shown that early intervention to teach children better self-control and coping skills is often more effective than trying to change behavior patterns that are established, so family-based programs often show positive results. Teenagers may need help with basic academic skills and social skills to improve communication. Methods of resisting drugs must be provided and reinforced. Drug recovery programs can be helpful but are often too expensive or not available for those who need them.

Indicators of substance abuse

Many people with substance abuse (alcohol or drugs) are reluctant to disclose this information, but there are a number of indicators that are suggestive of substance abuse:

Physical signs	Other signs
Needle tracks on arms or legs.	Odor of alcohol/marijuana on clothing
Burns on fingers or lips.	or breath.
Pupils abnormally dilated or constricted,	Labile emotions, including mood
watery eyes.	swings, agitation, and anger.
Slurring of speech, slow speech.	Inappropriate, impulsive, and/or risky
Lack of coordination, instability of gait.	behavior.
Tremors.	Lying.
Sniffing repeatedly, nasal irritation.	Missing appointments.
Persistent cough.	Difficulty concentrating/short term
Weight loss.	memory loss, disoriented/confused.
Dysrhythmias.	Blackouts.
Pallor, puffiness of face.	Insomnia or excessive sleeping.
	Lack of personal hygiene.

Guidelines for helping smokers quit

The US Department of Health and Human Services guidelines for helping smokers quit includes the following information:
- Ask about and record smoking status at every visit.
- Advise all smokers to quit and explain health reasons why quitting is beneficial.
- Assess readiness to quit by questioning and if willing, provide resources. If patient is not willing, provide support and attempt to motivate the person to quit with information.
- Assist smokers with a plan that sets a date (within 2 weeks), removes cigarettes, enlists family and friends, reviews past attempts, and anticipates challenges during the withdrawal period. The nurse practitioner must give advice about the need for abstinence and discuss

the association of smoking with drinking. Medications to help control the urge to smoke (patches, gum, lozenge, prescriptions) and resources should be provided.

- Follow-up monitoring should be done to evaluate progress and reinforce the program.

Bereavement

Bereavement occurs after the death of family, friend, or someone to whom a person identifies closely. It is a time of mourning and is part of the natural grieving process, but some people are not able to move past the grieving discuss process and may suffer signs related to depression, such as poor appetite, insomnia, and other symptoms, such as chest pain, that may mimic physical illnesses. Some may enter a stage of denial or anger that interferes with their daily activities and work. People suffering bereavement may present with vague and varied complaints. A careful history is important. Treatment varies according to the needs of the individual. In some cases, selective serotonin reuptake inhibitors (SSRIs) (such as Prozac® [fluoxetine]) may provide temporary relief, but the patient should be referred for psychological counselling, bereavement services, or psychiatric care, depending upon the severity of symptoms.

Exercise

Daily exercise is an important component of good health practices but should be age-appropriate, and some health conditions may pose restrictions. Toddlers and young children usually get exercise by running and playing and do not need organized activities, but others benefit from planned exercise:

- 4-5 year olds may participate in dancing, skating and other supervised activities but lack coordination and judgment about safety.
- 6-12 year olds are still growing and muscles are short, so they do best with non-competitive sports, such as bicycling and swimming, until about age 10. Team sports should be supervised to ensure children are not straining muscles. Weight lifting may be done at 11 to build strength. Gymnastics may begin but children should be monitored for eating disorders.
- 12-18 year olds can participate in any sports activity unless limited by illness or disability. Exercise should be done at least 3 times weekly for 30 minutes.
- Adults: Exercise should be done at least 30 minutes daily or 150 minutes/week.

Emergency contraception

Females who have had unprotected sexual intercourse, consensual or rape, are at risk for pregnancy and may desire emergency contraception. Emergency contraception inhibits ovulation and prevents pregnancy rather than aborting a pregnancy. Because the medications contain hormones (such as ethinyl estradiol and norgestrel or levonorgestrel) in differing amounts, this treatment is contraindicated in those with a history of thromboembolia or severe migraine headaches with neurological symptoms. The criteria for administration of emergency contraception include:

- ≤72 hours since unprotected sexual intercourse.
- Negative pelvic exam.
- Negative pregnancy test.

The regimen involves taking a first dose of 1-20 pills (depending upon the brand and concentration of hormones) and then a second dose of 1-20 pills 12 hours later. A follow-up pregnancy test should be done if the person does not menstruate within 3 weeks as the failure rate is about 1.5%. Side effects include nausea (relieved by taking medication with meals or with an antiemetic), breast tenderness, and irregular bleeding.

Preventing STDs

The Centers for Disease Control and Prevention (CDC) has developed 5 strategies to prevent and control the spread of sexually transmitted diseases (STDs):
- Educate those at risk about how to make changes in sexual practices to prevent infection.
- Identify symptomatic and asymptomatic infected persons who may not seek diagnosis or treatment.
- Diagnose and treat those who are infected.
- Prevent infection of sex partners through evaluation, treatment, and counseling.
- Provide pre-exposure vaccination for those at risk.

Practitioners are advised to obtain sexual histories of patients and to assess risk. The 5-P approach to questioning is advocated. One should ask about:
- Partners: Gender and number.
- Pregnancy prevention: Birth control.
- Protection: Methods used.
- Practices: Type of sexual practices (oral, anal, vaginal) and use of condoms.
- Past history of STDs: High-risk behavior (promiscuity, prostitution) and disease risk (human immunodeficiency virus [HIV]/hepatitis).

The Centers for Disease Control and Prevention (CDC) recommends a number of specific preventive methods as part of the clinical guidelines for prevention of sexually transmitted diseases (STDs):
- Abstinence/reduction in number of sex partners.
- Pre-exposure vaccination: All those evaluated for STDs should receive a hepatitis B vaccination, and men who have sex with men (MSM) and illicit drug users should receive hepatitis A vaccination.
- Male latex (or polyurethane) condoms should be used for all sexual encounters with only water-based lubricants used with latex.
- Female condoms may be used if male condom can't be used properly.
- Condoms and diaphragms should not be used with spermicides containing nonoxynol-9 (N-9) and N-9 should not be used as a lubricant for anal sex.
- Non-barrier contraceptive measures provide no protection from STDs and must not be relied on to prevent disease.
- Women should be counseled regarding emergency contraception with medication or insertion of a copper intrauterine device (IUD).

Mental health promotion at the community level

Mental health promotion at the community level focuses on helping people maintain optimal levels of health and wellbeing, providing preventive measures, and assessing risks and protective factors associated with mental health. Promotion efforts may include:
- Programs for children and adolescents, such as through mentoring or education, to help children learn coping and problem-solving skills.
- 12-step programs to help people maintain sobriety/abstinence through peer support.
- Early childhood intervention programs that help teach good parenting skills.

- Support programs for people with mental illness to help them learn skills needed to live independently.
- Sheltered workshops to provide opportunity for skill acquisition and employment for people with mental impairment.
- Anti-bullying campaigns targeting all ages.
- Programs to support the LGBT community and prevent abuse and prejudice.
- Senior citizens' programs to provide services and social activities.
- Primary, secondary, and tertiary preventive measures.
- Boys and girls clubs to promote social interaction in a safe environment.

Anticipatory guidance

Anticipatory guidance is a method of educating the patient and/or family about the diagnosis, prognosis, and future care. Anticipatory guidance allows patients and their parents/guardians to formulate realistic expectations with regards to the treatment plan. Anticipatory guidelines are a catalyst for bringing forth questions and concerns regarding patient development, treatment progress, disease progression, therapy outcomes, rehabilitation or palliation, and follow-up or community care. As with all communications, the nurse practitioner ensures anticipatory guidance is clear and concise by:
- Asking patients and/or families if they have any questions.
- Offering them a business card so they can phone with any questions they think of later.
- Giving written anticipatory guidance handouts so the patient and family have reference information available at home. Often, they will not retain verbal information due to the initial shock diagnosis and prognosis causes.
- Directing them to a reputable patient support group and arrange for the team's social worker to help them.
- Asking if they would like the chaplain to visit.

Usual anticipatory guidance vs. targeted anticipatory guidance

Usual anticipatory guidance is the practice of disseminating a generic set of guidelines to a certain patient population. For example, parents of a toddler may receive pamphlets and/or physician-directed education on milestones, socialization, toilet training, and discipline that are standard issue for the institution or catchment area. Targeted anticipatory guidance is when a healthcare provider specifically speaks to the individual questions and concerns of a patient and/or the parents/guardian. There are pros and cons to both types of guidance. For example, usual anticipatory guidance covers a larger spectrum of topics and concerns, but may not touch on the 1 troubling behavior that is of specific concern to the parent, such as tantrums or combative behavior. Targeted anticipatory guidance covers 1 concern thoroughly, but fails to provide guidance on other topics that may become concerns in the interim before their next visit.

Children/families

Providing anticipatory guidance to children/families is an important role for the nurse practitioner, who is guided by knowledge about risk factors and growth and development. As the child moves from 1 stage of development to another, the nurse should provide information first to the parents and then to the parents and child about what to expect in terms of development, both physically and emotionally, as well as how to minimize risk factors. Guidance may be related to a number of different areas of concern:

- Diet and nutrition, especially for those children at risk for obesity or eating disorders.
- Safety measures, including information about common types of childhood injuries.
- Sexual development and normal related changes and behaviors.
- Sports activities and exercise that is age-appropriate.
- General growth and development.
- Academic progress and advice about testing and intervention for learning disabilities.
- Peer influence.
- Drug and alcohol abuse.

Early adolescence

Children during early adolescence (11-14) are undergoing many changes in their bodies and emotions. Relationships with family and peers may begin to change, and children may be very self-conscious and concerned that they are normal. Anticipatory guidance helps children to navigate changes in their lives and to negotiate changes in relationships as they seek more autonomy:

- **Physical changes**: Outline what children should expect in terms of bodily changes, such as development of secondary sexual characteristics, including normal variations, and height and weight changes.
- **Cognitive changes**: Allow children to express changes in thought patterns and awareness and discuss how that relates to developing maturity and stress the importance of maintaining academic responsibilities.
- **Socio-behavioral changes**: Ask children about peer groups and pressures at school and discuss methods to avoid gangs, tobacco, drugs, alcohol, and abusive relationships.

Middle adolescence

Middle adolescence (15-17) is a time of conflict for many young people as they strive to establish an identity separate from their parents and at the same time fit in and find acceptance with their peers. For many, this is the most difficult time of adolescence, and the nurse practitioner should provide anticipatory guidance to the adolescent through this time, even if the adolescent appears uninterested. Adolescents want respect and often respond when treated with respect. Encouraging the adolescent to discuss issues is more productive than providing direct guidance:

- **Physical changes**: Discuss the responsibilities that come with sexual maturity, including abstinence or birth control. Demonstrate breast and testicular self-examinations.
- **Cognitive changes**: Discuss future goals including both life plans and academic plans, and also provide guidance in relation to the necessary steps the adolescent needs to take in order to meet those goals.
- **Sociobehavioral changes**: Discuss relationships and risk-taking behavior while focusing on means to increase safety.

Grief, mourning, and bereavement

Grief is a normal response to loss, and older adults may face the loss of spouse, family, income, status, health, mobility, home, and independence. Mourning is the public expression of grief, and bereavement is the time period of mourning. There are 3 primary types of grief:

- Acute: This occurs immediately in response to some type of loss and may be expressed as sadness, anger, fear, and anxiety.
- Anticipatory: This occurs when people fear a loss, such as the impending death of a spouse or transfer to a long-term care facility.
- Chronic grief occurs when people are not able to come to terms with loss, so grieving and mourning are prolonged, sometimes for years. People may develop anorexia, insomnia, panic attacks, self-destructive behaviors (alcohol and substance abuse), and contemplate or carry out suicide.

Chronic grief poses a serious risk to people and should be treated as depression, with antidepressants, psychological evaluation, and counseling.

Kübler-Ross's stages of grief

Grief is a normal response to the death or severe illness/abnormality of a patient. How a person deals with grief is very personal, and each will grieve differently. Elisabeth Kübler-Ross identified **5** stages of grief in *On Death and Dying* (1969), which can apply to both patients and family members. A person may not go through each stage but usually goes through 2 of the 5 stages:

- Denial: Patients/families may be resistive to information and unable to accept that a person is dying or impaired. They may act stunned, immobile, or detached and may be unable to respond appropriately or remember what's said, often repeatedly asking the same questions.
- Anger: As reality becomes clear, patient/families may react with pronounced anger, directed inward or outward. Women, especially, may blame themselves and self-anger may lead to severe depression and guilt, assuming they are to blame because of some personal action. Outward anger, more common in men, may be expressed as overt hostility.
- Bargaining: This involves if-then thinking (often directed at a deity): "If I go to church every day, then God will prevent this." The patient or family may change doctors, trying to change the outcome.
- Depression: As the patient and family begin to accept the loss, they may become depressed, feeling as if no one understands, and overwhelmed with sadness. They may be tearful or crying and may withdraw or ask to be left alone.
- Acceptance: This final stage represents a form of resolution and often occurs outside of the medical environment after months. Patients are able to accept death/dying/incapacity. Families are able to resume their normal activities and lose the constant preoccupation with their loved one. They are able to think of the person without severe pain.

Beliefs and traditions regarding death

Individual beliefs and traditions regarding death vary widely, and these affect how the patient and family deal with the end of life. The nurse practitioner should discuss these issues with the patient and/or family in order to ensure their needs are met. Those with strong spiritual beliefs may want spiritual advisors (priests, shamans, ministers, monks) present to provide support or perform rituals. People who have no belief in an afterlife may face death with resolution or may be frightened at the thought of the total end of their existence. Those who believe in reincarnation may find comfort in the thought of their rebirth but may also fear karma for the mistakes they made in this life. Some people believe in a loving God and others a vengeful God, so some may feel that they will be in a loving place after death while others fear they will suffer torment for their sins. The nurse practitioner should remain supportive and allow patients and families to express their feelings, fears, and concerns.

Supporting families of dying patients

Families of dying patients often find themselves in desperate need of adequate support from nursing staff that, unfortunately, often are unprepared for dealing with their grief and unsure of how to provide comfort. Some examples of support nursing staff can provide to families before death include:

- Stay with the family and sit quietly, allowing them to talk, cry, or interact if they desire.
- Avoid platitudes, "His suffering will be over soon."
- Avoid judgmental reactions to what family members say or do and realize that anger, fear, guilt, and irrational behavior are normal responses to acute grief and stress.
- Show caring by touching the patient and encouraging family to do the same.
- Note: Touching hands, arms, or shoulders of family members can provide comfort, but follow clues regarding touching provided by the family.
- Provide referrals to support groups if available.

The family requires much support when the patient dies:
- Time of death:
  o Reassure family that all measures have been taken to ensure the patient's comfort.
  o Express personal feeling of loss, "She was such a sweet woman, and I'll miss her" and allow family to express feelings and memories.
  o Provide information about what is happening during the dying process, explaining death rales, Cheyne-Stokes respirations, etc. Alert family members to imminent death if they are not present.
  o Assist to contact clergy/spiritual advisors.
  o Respect feelings and needs of spouse, children, and other family.
- After death
  o Encourage parents/family members to stay with the patient as long as they wish to say goodbye.
  o Use the patient's name when talking to the family.
  o Assist family to make arrangements, such as contacting funeral home.
  o If an autopsy is required, discuss with the family and explain when it will take place.
  o If organ donation is to occur, assist the family to make arrangements. Encourage family members to grieve and express emotions. Send card or condolence note if appropriate.

Primary, secondary, and tertiary prevention

Gerald Caplan's (1964) model for prevention in mental health includes three types of preventive measures:
- Primary: The focus is on helping people to cope with stress and decreasing stressors in the environment, specifically targeting at-risk groups. Examples include teaching parenting skills to parents; providing support services to the unemployed; providing food, shelter and

other services to the homeless; and teaching about the harmful effects of drugs and alcohol to schoolchildren.
- Secondary: The focus is on identifying problems early and beginning treatment in order to shorten the duration of the disorder. Examples include follow-up for patients at risk for recurrence, staffing rape crisis centers, providing suicide hotlines, and referrals as needed.
- Tertiary: The focus is on preventing complications and promoting rehabilitation through teaching patients socially-appropriate behaviors. Examples include teaching the patient to manage daily living skills, monitoring effectiveness of outpatient services, and referring patients to support services.

Visualization to reduce anxiety and promote healing

There are a number of methods used for visualization to reduce anxiety and promote healing. Some include audiotapes with guided imagery, such as self-hypnosis tapes, but the patient—even a child—can be taught basic techniques that include:
- Sit or lie comfortably in a quiet place away from distractions.
- Concentrate on breathing while taking long, slow breaths.
- Close the eyes to shut out distractions and create an image in the mind of the place or situation desired.
- Concentrate on that image, such as of a favorite place or activity, engaging as many senses as possible and imaging details.
- If the mind wanders, breathe deeply and bring consciousness back to the image or concentrate on breathing for a few moments and then return to the imagery.
- End with positive imagery.

Sometimes, patients are resistive at first or have a hard time maintaining focus, so guiding them through visualization for the first few times can be helpful.

Social support system

The family is integral to the social support system of the patient, but social support can come from a number of other sources:
- Friends: Friends often assume the supportive role of family, especially in modern society when family members may not live in close proximity.
- Governmental agencies: Medicare and Medicaid may provide support as well as Social Services for welfare assistance.
- Religious/spiritual advisors: Religion or spiritual beliefs provide comfort to many, and some patients may receive not only spiritual support but also concrete support, such as housing or other assistance, from religious institutions.
- Community agencies: Many different agencies, such as Meals-on-Wheels, senior citizen centers, and outreach programs may provide practical assistance.
- Self-help programs: 12-step programs (such as Alcoholics Anonymous (AA), Overeaters Anonymous (OA), and Narcotics Anonymous (NA)) and other self-help programs provide an ongoing support system for those seeking recovery.
- Internet: Increasingly, people are turning to message boards and social networking sites for support although there are always some risks involved in anonymous interactions.

Family Systems Theory

Bowen's Family Systems Theory suggests that one must look at the person in terms of his/her family unit because the members of a family have different roles and behavioral patterns, so a change in 1 person's behavior will affect the others in the family. There are 8 interrelated concepts:

- Triangle theory: Two people comprise a basic unit, but when conflict occurs, a third person is drawn into the unit for stability with the resulting dynamic of 2 supporting 1 or 2 opposing 1. This, in turn, draws in other triangles.
- Self-differentiation: People vary in need for external approval.
- Nuclear family patterns: marital conflict, 1 spouse dysfunctional, 1 or more children impaired, and emotional distance.
- Projection within a family: Problems (emotional) passed from parent to child.
- Transmission (multigenerational): Small differences in transmission from parent to child.
- Emotional isolation: Reducing or eliminating family contact.
- Sibling order: Influence on behavior and development.
- Emotional process (society): Results in regressive or progressive social movements.

Coerced treatment

Coerced treatment should be avoided if at all possible. However, many times patients who are suffering from mental illness may refuse medications or other treatments. These patients may be suffering from delirium, dementia, or psychosis. Patients who are admitted on a voluntary basis and are not violent towards themselves or others can legally refuse any treatment or medication. However, with patients that have been committed, certain criteria can justify coerced treatment. These criteria include the following:

- The patient is dangerous to themselves or others.
- Those administering treatment truly believe that the treatment has a good chance of helping the patient.
- The patient has been determined to be incompetent to make informed decisions.

Many times a positive therapeutic relationship between the nurse practitioner and the patient can help avoid the refusal of treatments. Patients may be willing to take medications in a different form, mixed in food, or at a different time.

Violence and aggression

Violence and aggression are commonly seen in the psychiatric and mental health population. The nurse practitioner must be aware of signs of impending violence or aggression in order to intervene.

- Violence is a physical act perpetrated against an inanimate object, animal, or other person with the intent to cause harm. Violence often results from anger, frustration, or fear and occurs because the perpetrators believe that they are threatened or that their opinion is right and the victim is wrong. Violence may occur suddenly without warning or following aggressive behavior. Violence can result in death or severe injury if the patient attacks a fellow patient or staff member.

- Aggression is the communication of a threat or intended act of violence and will often occur before an act of violence. This communication can occur verbally or non-verbally. Gestures, shouting, speaking increasingly loudly, invasion of personal space, or prolonged eye contact are examples of aggression requiring the patient be redirected or removed from the situation.

Characteristics of a crisis

A crisis occurs when a person is faced with a highly stressful event and the usual problem solving and coping skills fail to be effective in resolving the situation. This even usually leads to increased levels of anxiety and can bring about a physical and psychological response. The problem is usually an acute event (such as a death in the family, loss of employment, or divorce) that can be identified. It may have occurred a few weeks or even months before or immediately prior to the crisis and can be an actual event or a potential event. The crisis state usually lasts less than 6 weeks with the individual then becoming able to utilize problem-solving skills to cope effectively. A person in crisis does not always have a mental disorder; however, during the acute crisis, social functioning and decision making abilities may be impaired.

Situational crisis

The second type of crisis (in addition to developmental) is the situational crisis. This type of crisis can occur at any time in life. There is usually an event or problem that occurs and leads to a disruption in normal psychological functioning. These types of events are often unplanned and can occur with or without warning. Some examples that may lead to a situational crisis include the death of a loved one, divorce, unplanned or unwanted pregnancy, onset or change in a physical disease process, job loss, or being the victim of a violent act. The patient may feel completely overwhelmed, helpless, and unable to think clearly or act appropriately, causing feelings of shame and guilt. Some may experience denial. Events that affect an entire community can also cause individual and community situation crisis. Terrorist attacks or weather-related disasters, such as floods or tornadoes, are examples of events that can affect an entire community.

Developmental crisis

There are basically 2 different types of crises: developmental or maturational crisis and situational crisis. A developmental crisis can occur during maturation when an individual must take on a new life role. This crisis can be a normal part of the developmental process. A youth may need to face the crisis and resolve it to be able to move on to the next developmental stage. A developmental crisis may occur during the process of moving from adolescence to adulthood. Situations that could lead to developmental crisis include graduating from school, going away to college, or moving away from the parents' home. These situations would cause the individual to face a maturing event that requires the development of new coping skills.

Crisis management

Modern crisis theory originated with Dr. Erick Lindermann in the 1940s when he observed similar responses in survivors of the Cocoanut Grove fire that killed almost 500 people. He later established a mental health program with Dr. Gerald Caplan, who outlined the basis of crisis theory. Caplan believed that a crisis occurs when changes alter one's personal view of self and relationships with others. Caplan divided crises into those that were developmental and accidental (also referred to as situational). He further demonstrated that those who immediately had psychiatric help to deal with crises experienced better outcomes. Erik Erickson built on this concept of developmental crises by outlining the developmental stages through the lifetime, with each stage constituting a type of developmental crisis because failure to accomplish the goals at each stage can result in negative consequences.

Crisis intervention

The first step in crisis intervention is a thorough evaluation and assessment of the problem and the triggering event as well as assessment of risks, such as suicide. A plan should be devised in collaboration with the patient, taking resources into consideration. Steps in intervention include:
- Helping the patient to gain understanding about the cause of the crisis.
- Encouraging the patient to freely express thoughts and feelings.
- Teaching the patient different coping mechanisms and adaptive behaviors.
- Encouraging social interaction.

Crisis intervention usually requires 4 to 6 weeks. Social and cultural influences can greatly affect the ability and ways in which people deal with and work through crisis. People may have preconceived ideas and beliefs about asking for and accepting assistance from others. It is very important to consider the age of the individual when assessing the need for particular crisis interventions. The needs of an elderly adult will be different than those needs of a child.

Group therapy

Groups can be classified according to form:
- Homogeneous: Members chosen on a selected basis, such as abused women.
- Heterogeneous: An assortment of individuals with different diagnoses, ages, genders.
- Mixed: A group which shares some key features, such as the same diagnosis but differs in age or gender.
- Closed: A group in which new members are excluded.
- Open: A group in which the members and leaders change.

Types of groups according to purpose include:
- Task: Emphasis on achieving a particular assignment.
- Teaching: Developed to inform, such as teaching the rules of the unit.
- Supportive/Therapeutic: Assisting those who share the same experience to learn mechanisms to cope with trauma and to overcome the problem, such as a group for battered women.
- Psychotherapy: Helping the client reduce psychological stress by modifying behavior or ideas.

Tuckman's group development stages

Tuckman's (1965) group developmental stages include:
- Forming: Group director takes more of an active role while members take their cues from the leader for structure and approval. The leader lists the goals and rules and encourages communication among the members.
- Storming: This stage involves a divergence of opinions regarding management, power, and authority. Storming may involve increased stress and resistance may occur, as shown by the

absence of members, shared silence, and subgroup formation. At this point, the leader should promote and allow healthy expression of anger.

- **Norming:** It is at this stage where members express positive feelings toward each other and feel deeply attached to the group.
- **Performing:** The leader's input and direction decreases and mainly consists of keeping the group on course.
- **Mourning:** This is most deeply felt in closed groups when discontinuation of the group nears and in open groups when the leader or other members leave.

Gestalt therapy

The major concepts of Gestalt therapy, according to Perls, include:
- Therapy involves the removal of masks and facades.
- A creative interaction between the client and the therapist needs to be developed so the client can gain an ongoing awareness of what is being felt, sensed, and thought.
- Boundary disturbances may be described as a lack of awareness of the immediate environment, including features such as:
  o Projection: The fantasy of what another person is experiencing.
  o Introjection: Accepting the beliefs and opinions of others without question.
  o Retroflection: Turning back on oneself that which is meant for someone else.
  o Confluence: Merging with the environment.
  o Deflection: A method of interfering with contact, used by receivers and senders of messages.
- The goal of therapy is the integration of self and world awareness.

In Gestalt therapy, a number of techniques are used as part of the therapeutic process:
- Playing the projection: Stating an observation first about another person and then applying the same statement to oneself to learn about projecting feelings about the self onto others.
- Making the rounds: Speaking or doing something to other group members to experiment with new behavior.
- Completing sentence: "I take responsibility for…"
- Exaggerating a feeling or action: Clarifying the purpose or intent.
- Mirroring: Group member does role playing and then volunteers from the group do alternative role playing while the original role player observes.
- Empty chair dialoguing: Having an interaction with an imaginary provocateur in an empty chair.
- Taking the hot seat: Group member sits across from the leader and describes a personal problem with input by other team members on request of the leader.
- Role playing the dream world: Describing and playing parts of a dream.

Hogarth's techniques for family therapy

Hogarth's (1993) techniques in family therapy include:
- Joining: Finding and matching commonalities among family behaviors, while respecting their values.
- Gathering data: Completing a family history about the parents' original relationship and progressing to each family member in chronological order. A completed family "genogram" delineates significant relationships and events extending over 3 generations of the family.

- Encouraging interactions and relationships: Beginning with a family member discussing an issue important to the family, the therapist then clarifies and explains the family's communication. Each individual should be allowed to speak and express their feelings instead of allowing others to speak for them. Family members are then asked to share responsibility for resolution of problems instead of placing blame.

Albert Ellis' Rational Emotive Therapy

Key concepts of Albert Ellis' Rational Emotive Therapy include:
- People control their own destinies and interpret events according to their own values and beliefs.
- A-B-C theory: Activating event, belief, consequences (emotional and/or behavioral).
- Forms of irrational beliefs:
  o Something should be different.
  o Something is awful or terrible.
  o One cannot tolerate something.
  o Something or someone is damned or cursed.
- "Musturbatory" ideologies have 3 forms:
  o I must do well and win approval or I am a rotten person.
  o You must act kindly toward me or you are a rotten person.
  o My life must remain comfortable or life hardly seems worth living.
- Therapy consists of detecting and eradicating irrational beliefs:
  o Disputing: Detecting irrationalities, debating them, discriminating between logical and illogical thinking, and defining what helps create new beliefs.
  o Debating: Questioning and disputing the irrational beliefs.
  o Discriminating: Distinguishing between wants and needs, desires and demands, and rational and irrational ideas.
  o Defining: Defining words and redefining beliefs.

Richard Bandler and John Grinder's neurolinguistics programming

The major concepts of neurolinguistic programming (NLP) according to Bandler and Grinder include:

Representational systems	Sensory models by which people access information (audio, visual, kinesthetic).
Cues to representational systems	Preferred predicated: "View" that suggests a visual system. Eye-Accessing cues: Looking upward suggests a visual system. Hand movements: Pointing toward the ear suggests an auditory system. Breathing patterns: Suggest a kinesthetic system. Speech patterns/tones: Suggest an auditory system.
Language structure	Surface structure: Sentences native language speakers speak and write. Deep structure: Linguistic representations from which the surface structures of a language are derived. Ambiguity: A surface language may represent more than 1 deep structure.

Human modeling (representing through language)	Generalization: Specific experiences representing the entire category of which they are a member. Deletion: Selected portions of the world are exclud-ed from the representation created by an individ-ual. Distortion: Relationship among the parts of the model that differ from the relationships they were supposed to represent.

Aaron Beck's Cognitive Therapy

Aaron Beck discovered that during psychotherapy patients often had a second set of thoughts while undergoing "free association." Beck called these "automatic" thoughts, which were labeled and interpreted according to a personal set of rules. Beck called dysfunctional automatic thoughts "cognitive disorders." The key concepts in Beck's cognitive therapy include:

Therapist/client relationship	Therapy is a collaborative partnership. The goal of therapy is determined together. The therapist encourages the client to disagree when appropriate.
Process of therapy	Therapist explains: The perception of reality is not reality. The interpretation of sensory input depends on cognitive processes. Client taught to recognize maladaptive ideation, identifying: The observable behavior. The underlying motivation. His/her thoughts and beliefs. The client practices distancing the maladaptive thoughts and explores his/her conclusions and tests them against reality.
Conclusions	The client makes the rules less extreme and absolute, drops false rules, and substitutes adaptive rules.

Psychotherapeutic options for phobias

Psychotherapeutic interventions for patients with phobias include:
- Psychodynamic: awareness therapy to resolve childhood conflicts and to find healthy ways to deal with anxiety.
- Behavior therapy: has been found to be the most effective treatment, and includes:
  - Systematic desensitization:
    - Patient grades anxiety-provoking stimuli from the least to the most terrifying.
    - Patient taught to enter a relaxed state.
    - Maintaining relaxed state, patient envisions each anxiety-provoking stimulus, starting with the least fearful.
    - When desensitized to 1 stimulus, patient then moves up the list until the list is completed.
    - Patient then puts into practice the relaxation techniques when encountering a phobia stimulus outside the therapist's office.
  - Flooding: Intensive exposure to stimulus through imagery until fear can no longer be felt.

Interviewing substance-abusing patients

Issues to discuss with a substance-abusing patient during an initial interview include:
- Drug(s) and/or drink of choice: Amount, frequency and duration of use, route of administration, and when last used.
- The use of any other substances.
- Any history of and response to withdrawal.
- Any history of delirium tremens (DTs), seizures, blackouts, alcoholic amnesia, or past events of injury to self or others.
- Changes in mood and/or behavior.
- Sleep pattern changes.
- Eating habits and any associated changes.
- Problems with relationships, finances, legal system, occupation, school, family, medical disorders, and psychiatric disorders.
- Any family history of drug or alcohol use and mental health disorders.
- Access to substances of abuse.
- Previous substance abuse treatments.
- Longest period of being substance-free.

Interviews with family members and/or significant others may be warranted if denial or rationalization is suspected.

Psychotherapeutic and family therapy interventions used with OCD

Psychotherapeutic and family therapy interventions used with obsessive-compulsive disorder (OCD) patients include therapy oriented to develop expression of thoughts and impulses in a manner that is appropriate:

Behavioral therapies (which appear to have the greatest success):
- Combined exposure with training to delay obsessive responses. Best used in conjunction with pharmacotherapy.
- Steady decrease of rituals by exposure to anxiety-producing situations until patient has learned to control the related obsessive compulsion.
- Reducing obsessive thoughts by the use of reminders or noxious stimuli to stop chain-of-thought patterns, such as snapping a rubber band on the wrist when obsessive thoughts occur.

Family therapy (Primary issues):
- Attempts to avoid situations that trigger OCD responses.
- The tendency of family members to constantly reassure the patient (this is apt to support the obsession).
- Family therapy involves:
  o Remaining neutral and not reinforcing through encouragement.
  o Avoiding reasoning logically with patient.

Psychotherapeutic and family therapy interventions for panic disorders

Psychotherapeutic interventions:
- Psychodynamic: Therapy designed to help the family become aware of and to focus upon the origin of anxiety and develop tools to be able to resolve conflicts.
- Behavioral:
  - Education regarding origin of panic attacks.
  - Desensitization: using real or imagined phobic situations(s).
  - Reinforcement of self-control and relaxation techniques.
  - Patient must anticipate and be able to manage break-through symptoms.

Family dynamics and therapy:
- Patients with agoraphobia may require the presence of family members to be constantly in close proximity, resulting in marital stress and over-reliance on the children.
- Altered role performance of the afflicted member results in family and social situations that increase the responsibility of other family members.
- The family must be educated about the source and treatment of the disorder.
- The goal of family therapy is to reorganize responsibilities to support family change.

Psychotherapeutic therapy for dissociative fugue

Dissociative Fugue is characterized by sudden memory loss, moving to a new location, and adopting a new identity; it is not associated with head injury, substance abuse, or any other general medical condition. Therapy includes:
- Restoring memories and identity as soon as possible, sometimes under hypnosis.
- Identifying stressful events leading to the fugue.
- Identifying and treating any condition(s) caused by traumatic events. The trauma needs to be evaluated and resolved by allowing proper emotional expression in a safe environment.
- Hospitalizing if behavior becomes bizarre or injurious to self or others.
- Beginning marital therapy if the marital situation is stressful.
- Educating regarding stress management.

The family may be a source of stress, and family customs may forbid open and clear expression of anxiety and emotional pain. If family dynamics are a source of stress, family therapy is needed to improve interaction and problem solving. The family may need education to understand the patient's condition.

Psychotherapeutic interventions for PTSD for males and females

Psychotherapeutic interventions and treatment for post-traumatic stress disorder (PTSD) differ by gender because the recovery process needs to be tailored to the particular trauma. The purpose of individual therapy includes:
- Educating the patient that PTSD is caused by extraordinary stress rather than weakness.
- Ceasing to minimize the trauma.
- Dispelling inaccurate ideas the person may have about the illness.
- Minimizing or eliminating any shame they may feel about having PTSD.
- Constructing a new, caring relationship with oneself.
- Addressing the sleep problems often associated with PTSD.

Men respond to PTSD differently than females:
- They are generally unwilling to seek treatment.
- They tend to minimize the experience.
- Difficulties exist with male intimacy.
- Symptoms may manifest as aggression, substance abuse, or sexual dysfunction.
- Therapy for men should promote the expression of emotions.

Psychotherapeutic interventions for chronic pain disorder

Psychotherapeutic goals and interventions for patients with verified chronic pain disorder include:

Individual:
- Rehabilitate the patient so he/she can return to work.
- Teach the psychological consequences of acute or chronic pain.
- Educate the patient about relaxation techniques when pain frustration occurs.
- Educate patient on activities of daily living (ADLs) within parameters of pain limitations.
- Encourage exercise within the patient's limitations.

Family Dynamics/Therapy:
- Educate family members about acute and chronic pain.
- Educate family on how to respond to patient's pain.
- The roles and responsibilities of each family member may need to be reorganized to accommodate the patient's pain.

Group:
- Pain support groups.
- Exercise groups experiencing same type of pain.
- Pain management groups.
- Assertiveness and self-confidence support groups.

Behavior modification

Behavior modification is a type of systematic therapy that works toward the goal of replacing maladaptive behaviors with positive behaviors. This type of therapy can be utilized with individuals, groups, or entire communities. There are 3 types of behavioral modification:
- Operant conditioning utilizes positive reinforcement directed towards the desired behaviors. By utilizing positive reinforcement, the participant will want to repeat the good behaviors to gain the reward, creating a new pattern of operant conditioning can be effective with eating disorders, smoking cessation, or addictions.
- Desensitization, in which patients are increasingly exposed to those things that cause them stress (such as phobias) so that they can overcome their fears.
- Aversion therapy applies a negative consequence to an action (such as using medications to induce vomiting after drinking alcohol) to create negative associations with the action in order to modify behavior.

Dialectical behavioral therapy for BPD

Dialectical behavioral therapy was developed for treatment of those with borderline personality disorder (BPD). While accepting the patient, the nurse/therapist tries to help him/her change behavior by replacing dichotomous thinking that paints the world as black or white with rational (dialectical) thinking. This therapy is based on the premise that patients with BPD lack the ability to self-regulate, have a low tolerance for distress, and encounter social and environmental factors that impact their behavioral skills. Therapy includes:

- Cognitive behavioral therapy (weekly), focusing on adaptive behaviors that help the patient to deal with stress/trauma. Therapy focuses on a prioritized list of problems: suicidal behavior, behavior that interferes with therapy, quality of life issues, post-traumatic stress (PTS) response, respect for self, acquisition of behavioral skills, and patient goals.
- Group therapy (2.5 hours weekly) to help the patient learn behavioral skills such as self-distracting and soothing.

PTSD psychotherapy

Patients with post-traumatic stress disorder (PTSD) are usually treated with antidepressants, mood stabilizers, or antipsychotic drugs, depending on their symptoms, but therapy is essential. Some examples of PTSD therapy include:

- Cognitive-behavioral therapy (CBT): Patients learn to confront trauma through psychoeducation, breathing, imaginary reliving, and writing and are taught to self-monitor and recognize thoughts related to their trauma and method of coping, such as distraction and self-soothing.
- Eye-movement desensitization and reprocessing (EMDR): This form of CBT requires the patient to talk about the experience of trauma while keeping the eyes and attention focused on the therapist's rapidly moving finger. (There is no clear evidence this is more effective than standard CBT.)
- Family therapy: PTSD impacts the entire family, so counseling and classes in anger management, parenting, and conflict resolution may help reduce family conflict related to the PTSD.
- Sleep therapy: Patients may fear sleeping because of severe nightmares. Sleep therapy teaches methods to cope with nightmares through imagery rehearsal therapy and relaxation techniques.

Psychoeducation for bipolar disorder and schizophrenia

Psychoeducation, often part of cognitive behavioral therapy, involves teaching patients about their disease to help them manage symptoms and behavior:

- Bipolar disorder: Patients are taught to understand the patterns of their disease and the triggers of mood changes so they can seek appropriate medical help. Additionally, they are taught to use self-monitoring tools (ie, a daily record) to determine patterns of activity (ie, sleeping) so they can maintain a consistent schedule of eating, sleeping, and engaging in physical activities as consistency tends to reduce unstable mood swings.
- Schizophrenia: Patients must be taught about their disease and the effects of medications. Because medication may not eliminate all symptoms, such as hearing voices, patients are taught methods to test reality to determine if their perceptions are correct.

Codependency

Codependency is a condition that afflicts the "significant others" of an addict. Codependency and other maladaptive behaviors are learned so that each individual may survive in a stressful and emotionally painful environment. Codependent responses are typified by a desire to change the addict's behavior—the individual puts the other's needs before his or her own. Codependent individuals are often adult children of alcoholics and generally share the following characteristics: self-defeating; poor self esteem; seeking approval from others; fearing abandonment; and unable to express anger. A codependent individual attempts to meet other's needs at the expense of personal needs.

Strategies used in family therapy to manage addiction issues include:
- Evaluating the family system's level of denial, education, and insight.
- Refraining from blaming family members for the way they feel or act regarding codependency.
- Educating family members about chemical dependency and referral to alcoholics anonymous (AL-ANON) and/or alcoholics anonymous for teens (AL-ATEEN) for support.
- Supporting and reinforcing healthy change.

Complementary and alternative medicine

Complementary therapies are used as well as conventional medical treatment and should be included if this is what the patient/family wants, empowering the family to take some control. Complementary therapies vary widely and most can easily be incorporated into the plan of care. The National Center for Complementary and Alternative Medicine recognizes the following:
- Whole medical systems, including medical systems such as homeopathic, naturopathic medicine, acupuncture, and Chinese herbal medications.
- Mind-body medicine, including support groups, medication, music, art, or dance therapy.
- Biologically-based practices, including the use of food, vitamins, or nutrition for healing.
- Manipulative/body-based programs, including massage or other types of manipulation, such as chiropractic treatment.
- Energy therapies, including biofield therapies intended to affect the aura (energy field) that some believe surrounds all living things. These therapies include therapeutic touch and Reiki.
- Bioelectromagnetic-based therapies which use a variety of magnetic fields.

Aromatherapy & music therapy

Aromatherapy uses essential oils derived from plant extracts. These oils are applied topically to the skin, heated and inhaled, or sprayed in the environment. Practitioners believe that aromatherapy can be used to treat and prevent disease, but it is usually used as an adjunct and by itself is rarely harmful, although healing claims are dubious.

Music therapy involves listening to music (often classical but any music that the person likes is acceptable). Music therapy is most often used to reduce anxiety. It can also be used as part of visualization or meditation to help the person slow breathing and focus attention. Music is sometimes used as part of an exercise program to help the person pace the exercises. In this case, faster music may be used.

Ayurveda and traditional Chinese medicine

Ayurveda is a traditional Indian method of healing that focuses on balancing the mind, body, and spirit to prevent or cure illness. Practitioners believe that when the *prana* (life force) and basic metabolism (dosha) are out of balance, the person becomes ill. While people may still use Western medicines, they may also want to follow Ayurvedic traditions through the use of herbs, diet, special breathing exercises, and yoga. Because some herbs contain active ingredients found in medications, the nurse practitioner should ask about herbal supplements or dietary restrictions (often vegan). Traditional Chinese medicine (TCM) has some similarities to Ayurveda. TCM is concerned with balancing of the vital energy (Qi) of the body through diet, meditation, herbs, acupressure, acupuncture, and exercise, such as Tai Chi. Because TCM relies on the use of herbs, the nurse practitioner should ascertain which herbs are used.

Seclusion

Seclusion involves separating the patients from others by placing them in an environment from which they are unable to leave. In some cases, patients may just be taken to another room under supervision, but a typical seclusion room has padded walls, no furniture, and a locked door. Often there are no or only very small shatterproof windows. There is nothing in this environment that patients could utilize to injure themselves or someone else. Once patients have been placed in seclusion, they must be observed continuously to ensure that they do not harm themselves. This particular type of restraint is often viewed negatively, is associated with negative patient outcomes, and is rarely utilized as patients are usually medicated to control their behavior instead of secluded.

Restrictive measures

The use of restrictive measures is a last resort in most patient settings. Restrictive measures are utilized to promote patient safety. The most common type of restrictive measures includes physical restraints and seclusion. Every patient is entitled to being treated with the greatest personal respect and dignity. When a patient's activity is restricted, very careful monitoring is required. Specific documentation on the patient's well being should be performed per the facilities policy and usually includes a description of what occurred that led to restrictive measures and physical monitoring of the patient while in restraints. If restrictive measures have to be utilized, staff members should have attempted and documented any and all other attempts to de-escalate the situation. These restraint techniques should only be utilized during the time that the patient is considered dangerous to him/herself or others.

Restraint and seclusion of pediatric patients

Some consistent recommendations for the use of restraint and seclusion with pediatric patients, despite some variations in state, accrediting, and federal regulations, include:
- Using restraint and seclusion only as a last resort and only in cases where the patient and/or others are threatened.
- Maintaining time limits for restraint and seclusion:
  - Children ages 9 to 17 should be restrained and/or secluded no longer than 2 hours.
  - Children under the age of 9 should only be restrained and/or secluded for a maximum of 1 hour.
- Patients are released from restraint and/or seclusion as soon as it is healthy and safe to do so.

- Pressure and unsafe holds should not be applied to patients in restraints.
- Patients must be frequently monitored during the duration of the restraint and seclusion to ensure their safety and changes in behavior.

Restraints

Restraints are used to restrict movement, activity, and access. There are 2 primary types of restraints used with patients: clinical and behavioral. Behavioral restraints are more commonly used in the psychiatric unit or when patients are at risk of hurting themselves or others. More commonly, clinical restraints are used to ensure that the patient does not interfere with safe care. The federal government and the Joint Commission have issued strict guidelines for temporary restraints or those not part of standard care (such as post-surgical restraint):
- There must be a written policy.
- An assessment must be completed.
- An alternative method should be tried before applying a restraint.
- An order must be written.
- The least restrictive effective restraint should be used.
- The restraint must be removed, assessed, and findings documented at least every 2 hours.

Physical restraints may involve the use of a person physically restraining a patient or the use of a mechanical device to restrict movement.

Chemical restraints
Chemical restraints involve the use of medications, such as lorazepam or haloperidol, to manage a patient's behavior problems. This type of restraint is indicated when patients are extremely agitated or violent in order to prevent injury to themselves or others. Chemical restraints inhibit patients' physical movements and make their behavior more manageable. Medication used on an ongoing basis as part of treatment is not legally considered a chemical restraint, which is used only in emergent situations, even though the medications may be the same. There is little consensus about the use of chemical restraints although benzodiazepines and/or antipsychotics are frequently used to control severe agitation. Oral medications should be tried first before injections, as oral medication is less coercive. The trend in psychiatric medicine is to target medications to treat particular symptoms, such as severe agitation, rather than simply to chemically restrain the patient.

Criteria for psychiatric/mental health diagnoses

The standard references that provide criteria for making a mental health or psychiatric diagnosis include:
- North American Nursing Diagnosis Association (NANDA) is an association of professional nurses developed to standardize nursing terminology. In 2002, NANDA became NANDA International. Reference: North American Nursing Diagnosis Association. (1998-2000). *NANDA Nursing Diagnoses: Definitions and Classification.*
- The American Psychiatric Association produces the Diagnostic and Statistical Manual of Mental Disorders (DSM) through the work of task forces that study current research and practice in the field of psychiatry. The DSM-5 is the most current version, released May 2013.
- The World Health Organization produces the International Classification of Diseases to try to provide consistent diagnosis of disease worldwide: *International Classification of Diseases, Tenth Revision, Clinical Modification (2007) (ICD-10-CM)).*

Removal of the axial diagnosis system in the DSM-V

The multi-axial diagnostic system of DSM-IV comprised fives axes (or levels), with each axis representing a characteristic of mental disorders with some third-party reimbursement requiring that patients be evaluated in all five axes:
  I.   Clinical disorders: Major psychiatric disorders.
  II. Personality/Intellectual disabilities.
  III. General medical conditions.
  IV. Psychosocial and environmental problems.
  V.   Global Assessment of Functioning Scale (GAF).

DSM-V combines the first three axes into one category with severity rated along a continuum. Axes IV and V now require separate assessment with the GAF eliminated and practitioners advised to use other assessment instruments, such as WHODUS-2. Changes have occurred throughout the text. For example, "intellectual disability" has been replaced with "intellectual disability" and sub-types of schizophrenia have been eliminated. Autistic-associated disorders have been combined into one category, autism spectrum disorders. New additions include binge-eating disorder, disruptive mood dysregulation disorder, hoarding disorder, and excoriation (skin picking) disorder. The bereavement exclusion from depression has been removed.

Intellectual disability

Intellectual disability is usually diagnosed in patients <18 years of age. Patients may have difficulty adapting to changing environments, need guidance in decision-making, and have self-care or communication deficits. Behaviors range from shy and passive to hyperactive or aggressive. Those with associated physical characteristics (Down syndrome) or problems are often diagnosed early. Intellectual disability may be inherited (Tay-Sachs), toxin-related (maternal alcohol consumption), perinatal (hypoxia), environmental (lack of stimulation/neglect), or acquired (encephalitis, brain injury). Diagnosis involves performance results from standardized tests along with behavior analysis. There are 4 MR classifications based on intelligence quotient (IQ):
  - 55-69 – mild (85%): Educable to about sixth grade level. May not be diagnosed until adolescence. Usually able to learn skills and be self-supporting but may need assistance and supervision.
  - 40-54 – moderate (10%): Trainable and may be able to work and live in sheltered environments or with supervision.
  - 25-39 – severe (3-4%): Language usually delayed and can learn only basic academic skills and perform simple tasks.
  - <25 – profound (1-2%): Usually associated with neurological disorder with sensorimotor dysfunction. Require constant care and supervision.

Brain waves

Brain waves, originating in the cerebral cortex, represent fluctuating changes in the electrical activity of the extracellular fluid in the brain. Waves may be recorded on an open exposed brain with an electrocorticogram (ECoG) or on the outside of the head with an electroencephalogram (EEG). Wave patterns include:
  - Alpha: Recorded from the posterior portion head with a frequency of 3 to 18 cycles/second, alpha waves occur when the person is awake but resting with eyes closed but disappear when the person sleeps or opens the eyes.

- 123 -

- Beta: Recorded from the anterior portion of the head with a frequency of >13 cycles/second, beta waves occur during periods of mental activity or stress.
- Theta: Recorded from the parietal and temporal areas with a frequency of 4 to 7 cycles/second, theta waves are common in children but usually only occur in some adults during times of acute stress or during the first stages of sleep.
- Delta: Originating in the cerebral cortex with a frequency <4 cycles/second, *delta* waves occur during sleep.

ADHD

Attention-deficit/hyperactivity disorder (ADHD) is commonly diagnosed in pre-school or school-aged children, although some are diagnosed as adults. It is more common in males than females. The person may have constant inattentiveness, display unruly conduct, and exhibit antisocial behaviors. ADHD is characterized by hyperactivity-impulsiveness and inattention, with some primarily hyperactive-impulsive, some inattentive, and some combined. ADHD may be delayed in its diagnosis. Behaviors may persist through adolescence and appear in some form into adulthood with less impulsivity as the child ages. Diagnostic criteria include:
- ≥6 symptoms of inattention or ≥6 symptoms of hyperactivity-impulsivity, inappropriate for developmental level persisting for ≥6 months.
- Presence of symptoms prior to age 7.
- Symptoms present in ≥2 settings (home, school, work, play).
- Significant impairment socially, academically, and/or occupationally.
- Not exclusively related to other disorder (schizophrenia, mood disorder).

Treatment for ADHD is long-term and involves both the patient and the family. Treatment may include pharmacotherapy, psychotherapy, behavioral therapy, social skills training, or support services.

Learning disorders

Children with learning disorders often fall substantially behind their peers in regards to expected skill and academic achievement levels. These disorders are often classified into verbal and non-verbal groups that include reading, writing, and mathematics. Dyslexia, a reading disorder, is not defined by reduced intelligence. It has both genetic and environmental components and is a deficit involving the processing of the sounds involved in speech. Mathematic disorders appear to involve a dysfunction of the right hemisphere of the brain. Medical conditions, such as Turner's syndrome or seizure disorders, can lead to right hemispheric dysfunction. Diagnosis of these disorders is often not made until the child reaches school and experiences a decreased performance. This group can often have low self-esteem and may need support to assist with these issues. Specialized educational training can improve functioning.

Oppositional defiant disorder

Oppositional defiant disorder (ODD) means the patient has an abnormally intense disregard for authority figures, primarily parents or guardians. Behavior with ODD is less severe than with conduct disorder and usually does not involve aggressive behavior toward people, property, or animals. The ODD patient challenges authority figures because of learned behaviors, such as negative reinforcement. A pattern of mutual negative reinforcement occurs between patient and authority figure in such a manner that the patient confronts all requests with extreme defiance. The diagnostic criteria for ODD include a negative, hostile pattern of behavior persisting ≥6 months. The pattern may consist of having frequent loss of temper, arguing with authority figures, showing defiance, blaming others, and annoying others. The behavior is so aberrant as to cause problems at work, school, or play. The person with ODD exhibits social and academic impairment that are not the result of a psychotic or mood disorder.

Conduct disorder

Conduct disorder is characterized by a blatant disregard for other people's feelings and property, societal norms, and etiquette. Onset may be during childhood or adolescence. Conduct disorders may spring from interplay of the child's genotype with the environment, as illustrated in a stress-diathesis model. Conduct disorder likely develops when a patient has a genetic predisposition or weakness and experiences childhood stresses, such as abuse, peripartum stress, neglect, harsh parenting, or poverty. Patients who are predisposed to conduct disorder often develop psychosis, depression, violent mood swings, and irritability. Conduct disorder is more prevalent in males than females. The diagnostic criteria for conduct disorder requires a relentless pattern of behavior that shows a lack of respect for the rights of others as well as social norms. Indications include aggression to people or animals (bullying, abuse), destruction of property (fire-setting, destruction), deceitfulness or theft (including criminal acts), and serious violations of rules (defiance before age 13, truancy, running away).

Autism

Autism is 1 of several different types of pervasive developmental disorders (PDDs). These children, usually exhibiting symptoms within the first 2 years, are often isolated with an inability to socialize. Their communication abilities are limited. Autism is characterized by delay in social interactions with others, social use of language, or exercise of imagination in play. Diagnostic criteria include at least 6 of the following:
- Impairment of social interactions (in at least 2 areas): Inability to use/understand non-verbal communication, inability to establish peer relationships, lack of socialization skills, and inability to express emotions.
- Impairment of communication (In at least 1 area): Delay or lack of spoken language without attempt to compensate (e.g., through gestures), inability to carry out a conversation with others, repetitive use of language (echolalia), and inability to carry out make-believe play or imitation appropriate to developmental level.
- Restrictive repetitive or stereotyped behavior (in at least 1 area): Preoccupation with some behavior patterns (head banging, rituals), inflexibility, and/or preoccupation with objects.

Communication disorders

Communication disorders impair a person's ability to communicate with others through speech or language development. These disabilities often go unnoticed and lead to delays in social and educational development. Examples of communications disorders include:
- Expressive language disorder: Impaired language development with limited vocabulary and sometimes abnormal phonation.
- Mixed receptive-expressive language disorder: Combination of limited vocabulary and abnormal phonation, difficulty understanding words, and/or abnormal auditory processing.
- Phonological Disorder: Impairment in production of speech sounds with absence or substitution of sounds, causing interference with work, school, or social communication.

- Stuttering: Onset is usually at 2-7 years. Sometimes associated with tics, blinking, or other motor movements.

Because their speech may not sound as expected, patients may experience teasing or ridicule, leading to self-esteem problems and social isolation. Communication disorders may be related to intellectual disability, speech-motor deficit, hearing/sensory impairment, or environmental deprivation. Mild communication disorders may not be diagnosed until adolescence. Specialized educational training and speech therapy may help improve symptoms.

Rett's syndrome

Rett's syndrome is a pervasive developmental disorder in females, characterized by normal prenatal development, normal motor development in the first 5 months of life, and a normal head circumference. However, between 5-48 months of age, head growth decelerates and the loss of purposeful use of the hands, along with gait abnormalities, seizures, and intellectual disability appears.

Stage I (Early onset) Age 6-18 mo. Characteristics: The infant begins to exhibit less eye contact, diminished interest in playing, and delays in motor skill development (crawling and sitting).

Stage II (Rapid destruction) Age 1-4 yrs. Characteristics: Previously gained skills, such as use of hands and speech, are lost. Purposeless hand movements such as wringing, grasping or finger wriggling begin but disappear when child is asleep. Deceleration of head growth is usually evident.

Stage III (Pseudo-stationary) Age 2-10 yrs. Characteristics: Apraxia and seizures are prominent. A child may show more interest in her surroundings than she did during Stage II, and her alertness, attention span, and communication skills may improve. Many girls remain in this stage for most of their lives. Stage IV (Motor deterioration) Age ---→ Characteristics: Common features include: reduced mobility, muscle weakness, rigidity spasticity, dystonia, and scoliosis. Girls who were previously able to walk may stop walking. Generally, there is no decline in cognition, communication, or hand skills. Repetitive hand movements may decrease, and eye gaze usually improves

Asperger's disorder

Asperger's disorder is part of the autism spectrum but symptoms are less severe, and Asperger's disorder does not include impairment of language or cognitive development that is common in autism. Intellectual disability is usually not associated with Asperger's although some may exhibit mild retardation. Motor difficulties, such as clumsiness and awkward gate, may be evident. Many of those with Asperger's disorder also have attention-deficit/hyperactivity disorder (ADHD), and some develop depression. Social impairment, including inability to use/understand non-verbal behavior or to establish peer relationships, is common with behavior often considered eccentric. People with Asperger's may focus on 1 topic in a conversation, ignoring the input of others, and may be preoccupied with certain topics or activities to the exclusion of others. The disorder is usually not evident during the first 3 years, and some may learn compensating behavior by adolescence, but patients often have difficulty establishing friendships and may feel isolated.

Tourette's disorder

Tourette's disorder is a dominant genetic disorder characterized by motor and vocal tics. Boys are 3 times more likely to inherit it than girls, with onset usually during childhood or early adolescence. Girls with a Tourette's parent are more likely to manifest obsessive-compulsive disorder and attention-deficit/hyperactivity disorder (ADHD). Tourette's children are likely to have emotional problems because their barking, echolalia (repeating others' words), and coprolalia (loud cursing) stigmatizes them at school. Tourette's disorder is often associated with obsessive-compulsive behavior. Symptoms worsen around puberty and then may lessen. Criteria include:

- Both motor and vocal tics.
- Numerous tics daily or intermittently for >1 year with no tic-free period more than 3 consecutive months.
- Onset <18.
- Not a result of another disorder, such as Huntington's.

Tic disorders

Tics are sudden, involuntary, repetitive movements or sounds that appear out-of-context. Tics affect mostly Caucasian males and may be chronic or transient. Tics include uncontrollable blinking, grimacing, jerking, shrugging, barking, and obscene expletives. One-quarter of schoolchildren have transient tics lasting 4 weeks to 1 year. Tics are caused by blood flow problems through the basal ganglia and anterior cingulate cortex, and imbalance of dopamine, serotonin, and cyclic adenosine monophosphate (AMP). The cause is genetic in 75% of cases. Stroke, viral encephalitis, strep infection, and head trauma also cause tics. Tics often progress from the face, towards the neck and torso, to the feet. With support, many patients effectively manage tics throughout childhood, and the disorder remits in 73% of cases by adulthood. However, a childhood tic that worsens with age is likely to become a severe tic in adulthood. Ritalin, Cylert, antihistamines, amphetamines, tricyclic antidepressants, anticonvulsants, opioids, and cocaine worsen tics. Tics are often more manageable when the patient learns to effectively control their stress and anxiety.

Enuresis

Enuresis is repeated involuntary urinary incontinence in children old enough to have bladder control, usually about 5-6 years old. Diabetes and other disorders should be ruled out, although 95% are not associated with structural or neurological disorders. There are 3 types:

- Primary: The child has never been dry at night, and incontinence is associated with delay in maturation and small functional bladder rather than stress or psychiatric disorders.
- Intermittent: The child stays dry part of the time with episodes of incontinence at night.
- Secondary: The child has had long periods (6-12 months) staying dry and then is incontinent because of infection, stress, or sleep disorder.

Incontinence may occur only at night (most commonly in the first third of the night during rapid eye movement [REM] sleep), only during the day (uncommon after age 9), or during both day and night. Some children postpone urination for various reasons until they are incontinent. Criteria include involuntary urination ≥2 times weekly for ≥3 months or severe social/academic impairment.

Encopresis

Encopresis is the voluntary or involuntary passage of stool in places or manners that are inappropriate for a child, 80% of whom are male, 4 years or older. There are 2 types:

- Retentive: Accounts for about 80% of those affected and is characterized by a history of long-term, painful constipation and the development of overflow diarrhea. The chronic constipation causes distention of the rectum and stretching of both the internal and

- 127 -

external anal sphincters; as a result, the child may no longer feel the urge to defecate, so stool eventually leaks from the rectum, causing chronic fecal incontinence.
- Non-retentive: Accounts for the other 20%. Non-retentive encopresis, usually involving passage of normally formed stools on a daily basis, does not involve constipation or bowel abnormalities, except in a small subset that may have irritable bowel syndrome, but is generally a behavioral/psychological problem. When encopresis is deliberate, the child may have conduct disorder or oppositional defiant disorder.

Separation anxiety

Separation anxiety disorder is more severe than normal separation and stranger anxiety, which starts around the age of 7 months and persists into childhood. Separation anxiety disorder is excessive concern regarding separation from the principal caregiver, featuring:
- Safety concerns and excessive worry about being lost.
- Sleep disturbances, such as nightmares centered on the theme of separation and refusal to go to sleep.
- School refusal and reluctance to play with friends.
- Clinginess to family members.
- Psychosomatic complaints.
- Temper tantrums.
- Panic attacks.

These symptoms must last more than 4 weeks and cause functional impairment to be diagnosed as separation anxiety disorder. The exact cause of separation anxiety disorder is unknown. Environment, genotype, and family history all influence the development of separation anxiety disorder.

Delirium

Delirium is an acute sudden change in consciousness, characterized by reduced ability to focus or sustain attention, language and memory disturbance, disorientation, confusion, audiovisual hallucinations, sleep disturbance, and psychomotor activity disorder. Delirium differs from disorders with similar symptoms in that delirium is fluctuating. Delirium occurs in 10-40% of hospitalized older adults and about 80% of patients who are terminally ill. Delirium may result from drugs, such as anticholinergics, and numerous conditions, including infection, hypoxia, trauma, dementia, depression, vision and hearing loss, surgery, alcoholism, untreated pain, fluid/electrolyte imbalance, and malnutrition. Delirium increases risks of morbidity and death, especially if untreated. Diagnosis includes interview to identify triggers and history and chart review. Asking a patient to count backward from 20 to 1 and spell first name backward can identify attention deficit. Treatment includes providing a sitter to ensure safety and decreasing dosage of hypnotics and psychotropics. Medications to reduce symptoms include trazodone, lorazepam, and haloperidol.

Schizophrenia

<u>Initial symptoms</u>
Schizophrenia is a psychotic disorder characterized by personality disintegration and distortion in the perception of reality, thought processes, and social development. Criteria include:
- Presence of ≥2 of the following for a significant time during a one-month period: delusions, withdrawal, odd behavior, hallucinations, inability to care for self, disorganized speech, catatonia, alogia (inability to speak because of mental deficiency, mental confusion, or aphasia), and avolition (inability to initiate and persist in goal-directed behavior).
- Only 1 of the above symptoms if the following are present:
  o Bizarre delusions such as thought broadcasting or being controlled by a dead person.
  o Hearing a voice constantly commenting on a person's behavior or thoughts. The voice may be from God, Satan, a friend, or a relative. Patients experiencing these voices often attempt to quiet or eliminate the voices by turning the radio or television to static to drown out the voices.
  o Hearing 2 or more voices conversing with each other.
- Social and/or occupational dysfunction for a major portion of time since onset.

<u>Childhood schizophrenia</u>
Schizophrenia rarely presents in children and adolescents, but it can occasionally present early. Many symptoms of schizophrenia mirror normal childhood characteristics and fantasies, so it is particularly difficult to diagnose in this age group. Symptoms of early-onset schizophrenia include:
- Paranoia.
- Visual and/or auditory hallucinations.
- Bizarre thoughts and beliefs.
- Impaired or confused concentration, speech, and social skills.
- Inappropriate reaction to events.
- Developmental delays.

Children with schizophrenia will have disturbances in all settings and are unlikely to show interest in making friends with others. Hallucinations and delusions must persist beyond 6 months in duration and continue past the age of 7. Early-onset schizophrenia has a very poor prognosis. The patient is high risk for suicide and symptom-related accidental death.

<u>Ongoing symptoms</u>
Schizophrenia is a chronic disorder, so diagnosis requires continuous signs of disturbance for at least 6 months, including:
- At least 1 month of active symptoms, *and*
- Prodromal and residual phases that include the following symptoms:
  o Social isolation.
  o Catatonic behavior.
  o Unusual behavior, such as talking to oneself in public.
  o Little attention to personal hygiene.
  o Odd speech characterized by the following:
    ▪ Circumstantiality: Talking in circles around the issue.
    ▪ Tangentiality: Moving from 1 topic to another where the logical connection may be visible but is not relevant to the issue being discussed.
    ▪ Magical thinking: Including ideas or delusions of reference (such as having magical powers obtained from trees).
    ▪ Recurrent illogical perceptual experiences.

- 129 -

Schizophrenia is a related group of psychiatric illnesses that include the subtypes: paranoid, disorganized, catatonic, undifferentiated, and residual. Symptoms may vary widely but include positive symptoms, such as delusions and hallucinations, and negative symptoms, such as flat affect and lack of motivation. Co-morbidities, such as obsessive-compulsive disorder and depression, are common as well as substance abuse and suicidal tendencies. In older adults, psychosis often reduces, but some cognitive impairment is common during all ages and is a persistent problem with chronic schizophrenia. There are about 300,000 older adult schizophrenics in the United States and about two-thirds are in nursing homes but only 15,000 in psychiatric hospitals, suggesting that cognitive impairment is the bigger problem with older adults. Schizophrenia is treated with typical antipsychotics (chlorpromazine, haloperidol, loxapine) and atypical antipsychotics (olanzapine, clozapine, risperidone), which provide better reduction in negative symptoms. All are associated with significant side effects, including tardive dyskinesia, but atypical antipsychotics have fewer side effects, and studies suggest they may be better tolerated in older adults.

Subtypes

Subtypes of schizophrenia include:

- Paranoid schizophrenia: Characterized by developing delusions of persecution or personal grandeur, accompanied by auditory hallucinations.
- Disorganized schizophrenia: Characterized by a flat affect or an affect inappropriate for the situation, associated with bizarre mannerisms, and social isolation. Onset occurs early in life and often is persistent.
- Catatonic schizophrenia: Disturbances may be manifested by mannerisms, such as posturing, immobility, mutism, and negativism that may last for minutes or hours. In general, males experience their initial catatonic episode in their teens or 20s, while women usually experience first episodes in their 20s or early 30s.
- Undifferentiated schizophrenia: Meets general diagnostic conditions of schizophrenia but does not fit the criteria for other subtypes.
- Residual schizophrenia: Absence of hallucinations and delusions; however, 2 or more residual symptoms continue. Must be in absence of dementia or organic brain disease.

Schizoaffective disorder

Schizoaffective disorder is characterized by the initial symptoms of schizophrenia (delusions, hallucinations, disorganized speech and behavior, catatonia, negative symptoms) with delusions or hallucinations for at least 2 weeks out of a one-month period. The patient must experience a major depressive, major manic, or mixed episode. The symptoms must not be related to substance abuse. Auditory hallucinations are common before onset of depression. Subtypes of schizoaffective disorder include bipolar type (manic or mixed episodes) and depressive type (only depression). Schizoaffective disorder is less common than schizophrenia, and symptoms are usually less severe, but social and work activities dysfunction is common. Onset is usually in early adulthood. Differential diagnoses include delirium, dementia, schizophrenia, and mood disorders with psychosis.

PTSD

Post-traumatic stress disorder (PTSD) is an anxiety disorder that develops as a response to a severe emotional or physical trauma. The patient is typically numb at first but later has symptoms that may include excessive irritability, nightmares, flashbacks to the traumatic scene, and overreactions to sudden noises. PTSD typically develops after a terrifying ordeal that involved physical harm or the threat of physical harm, such as military combat, assault, rape, serious accidents, abuse, and natural disasters.

Feelings common to these traumatic experiences include:
- Overpowering terror, helplessness, and fear of being killed.
- Recurrent intrusive thoughts of trauma in dreams, during awake periods, or through persistent flashbacks.
- Avoidance of thoughts or recollections about the trauma.
- Avoidance of persons or situations that provoke the memory of the original trauma.
- Diminished interest in activities or persons.
- Increased startle reflex, sleep disturbances, outbursts of temper, and difficulty concentrating.

Phobias

A phobia is an uncontrollable, unfounded, and persistent fear of a specific object, situation, or activity that actually poses no threat. If confronted with the item causing the fear, anxiety, sweating and tachycardia may develop. In severe situations, a panic may develop. Specific phobias include a number of subtypes:
- Animals: Includes animals (such as dogs or cats) and insects (such as spiders) with onset usually during childhood.
- Natural environment: Includes fear of storms, water, and heights with onset usually during childhood.
- Blood-injection-injury: Includes fear of needles, blood.
- Situational: Includes fear of flying, tunnels, and bridges with onset in childhood or mid-20s.
- Other: Includes various phobias, such as fear of choking, falling, sounds.

Social phobias are characterized by fear of social or performance activities, resulting in anxiety and/or panic attacks, which the person recognizes as excessive but cause the person to avoid triggering situations. Onset is usually during adolescence and often occurs in those with history of shyness. Duration is >6 months in those <18 and may persist throughout life.

GAD

Generalized anxiety disorder (GAD) is an unrealistic apprehension and worry that persists for 6 or more months. GAD may be accompanied by tension, sweating, irritability, and hypervigilance. Symptoms include:
- Motor tension: Tremulousness, muscle tension.
- Autonomic arousal: Shortness of breath, tachycardia, dry mouth, and diarrhea.
- Vigilance: Insomnia and a feeling of being edgy.
- Depression.
- Impaired quality of life.

Levels of anxiety include:
- Mild: Slight physical arousal but retains the ability to learn well.
- Moderate: Physical symptoms are present.
- Severe: Physical symptoms interfere with day-to-day activities, difficulty concentrating, very anxious.

- Panic: Terrified, little-or-no ability to concentrate, shortness of breath, palpitations, fear of dying.

Panic disorder

Panic disorder is chronic, repeated, and unexpected panic attacks, with spells of overwhelming fear, apprehension, terror, and being in danger when there is no specific cause. Characteristics include:
- Panic attack often begins with rapidly increasing sense of tragedy, coupled with tachycardia, difficulty breathing, and diaphoresis.
- Episodes last from minutes to several hours and may include sense of unreality, detachment from oneself, fainting, vertigo, choking, and chest pain. Initial attacks usually occur in an anxiety-provoking situation, while successive attacks are spontaneous and unexpected.
- Those affected often report to the Emergency Department thinking that they may be having a "heart attack" or severe respiratory problems.
- Anticipatory anxiety may exist between attacks because of fear that another may occur without warning.
- Severity of attacks may range from minimal to severe with disabling symptoms.

Agoraphobia

Agoraphobia (literally "fear of the marketplace") can occur with or without panic disorder. Agoraphobia is fear and anxiety about being in a situation or place from which escape may be difficult, causing the person to avoid these places/situations. This often results in the person being unable to leave the home or to be in a crowd, elevator, bus, or other enclosed space. When associated with panic disorder, the combination of agoraphobia and panic attack is followed by ≥1 month of worry and anxiety about the possibility of recurrence, concern over implications of the attack, and avoidance behaviors related to preventing another attack. Agoraphobia without panic disorder is similar, although the concern is to avoid having embarrassing or panic-like attacks that are less acute than with panic disorder. To meet the diagnosis of agoraphobia, the disorder must not be related to substance abuse or another medical condition.

Major depressive disorder

A major depressive episode is a depressed mood, profound and constant sense of hopelessness and despair, or loss of interest in all or almost all activities for a period of at least 2 weeks. Family history of depression is a major risk factor. Developmental hormone changes at puberty or hormone disruption from disease can also contribute to depression. Depression is associated with neurotransmitter dysregulation, especially serotonin and norepinephrine. Major depression can be mild, moderate, or severe, and is characterized by a combination of symptoms that interfere with the ability to work, study, sleep, eat, and enjoy once pleasurable activities. Criteria include at least 5 of the following (including the first 2):
- Depressed mood most of the day.
- Diminished interest in most or all activities previously found enjoyable.
- Significant weight gain or loss without dieting.
- Insomnia or hypersomnia.
- Persistent pessimism.
- Constant fatigue.
- Feelings of worthlessness.
- Reduced ability to focus on tasks.

- Recurring thoughts of death or suicide.

Bipolar disorder

Bipolar disorder is a mood disorder characterized by mania, depression, or both. Subtypes include:
- Bipolar I: Characterized by at least 1 manic episode, sometime following an episode of depression. This form of bipolar usually includes cycling between mania and depression with episodes of psychosis that include paranoia and hallucinations.
- Bipolar II: Characterized by at least 1 episode of depression and at least 1 episode of hypomania (shorter lasting and less severe than mania) with the depressive periods of longer duration than hypomanic periods.
- Cyclothymia (Bipolar III): Characterized by milder mood swings.
- Bipolar not otherwise specified (NOS): Mood disorder without a clear pattern.

Some people with bipolar disorder may experience rapid cycling between depression and mania, often more than 4 times in a year, with mood changes occurring rapidly (within a few hours). Additionally, some people may experience a mixed type of bipolar disorder in which depression and mania both occur at the same time.

Manic episodes
Bipolar disorder is characterized by manic episodes alternating with depressive episodes that occur in varying patterns interspersed with periods of normal mood (euthymia). A manic episode is a distinct period characterized by extremely elevated mood, energy, and unusual thought patterns, causing impairment in occupational functioning and social activities for at least 1 week. Criteria include presence of at least 3 of the following during the same period:
- Unrealistic, grandiose beliefs about one's abilities or powers.
- Rapid and pressured speech.
- Racing thoughts, jumping quickly from 1 idea to the next.
- Looseness of thought patterns.
- Easily distracted and unable to concentrate.
- Feeling unusually "high" and optimistic.
- Increased interest in goal-directed activity.
- Acting recklessly without thinking about the consequences:
  o Questionable business transactions.
  o Wasteful expenditures of money.
  o Unsafe sexual activity.
  o Unusual social interactions.
  o Highly vocal arguments uncharacteristic of previous behaviors.
- Decreased need for sleep, but feeling extremely energetic.
- Delusions and hallucinations (in severe cases).

Depressive episodes
The symptoms of the depressive phase of bipolar disorder are the opposite of those symptoms that occur during the manic phase; additionally, suicide is a constant concern for those suffering through the depressive phase. Depressive episodes include:
- Feelings of hopelessness or helplessness.
- Putting affairs in order as if leaving somewhere.
- Acting recklessly as if not caring about one's life.
- Suicidal ideation: Seeking out weapons or pills that could be used to commit suicide.

- Loss of interest in enjoyable pastimes.
- Physical and mental sluggishness.
- Appetite or weight changes.
- Sleeping too much.
- Concentration and memory problems.
- Feelings of self-loathing, shame, or guilt.
- Ruminating about death, self-harm, or suicide.

Children and adolescents

Bipolar disorder is increasingly diagnosed in children and adolescents, but symptoms may vary from those of adults and may vary as the child's brain matures. Children often present with behavioral problems. Symptoms, usually after age 4, include:
- Violent rages, temper, hostility.
- Preoccupation with violence.
- Depressive periods or severe sadness.
- Pronounced separation anxiety.
- Inappropriate sexualized behavior.
- Suicidal ideation.
- Food/object cravings.
- Bossing, bullying behavior.
- Risk-taking behavior and grandiose beliefs.
- Delusions, hallucinations.
- Rapid speech, thoughts.
- Sleep disorders.

About 90% of all children diagnosed with bipolar disorder continue to experience the disorder throughout adulthood. However, early treatment during adolescence opens the door for remission. The bipolar child is high-risk for school failure, and 18% commit suicide.

Older adults

Bipolar disorder, a psychiatric affective disorder characterized by mood swings ranging from depression to mania, includes subtypes bipolar I, bipolar II, cyclothymia, rapid cycling, and mixed state. Co-morbid conditions include substance abuse, thyroid disorders, suicidal tendencies, obsessive-compulsive disorder, post-traumatic stress disorder, and dementia. Those with late onset (>50) tend to have less severe symptoms than those with early onset. Symptoms include severe mania, hypomania, normal mood, mild to moderate depression and severe depression. Symptoms may be precipitated by environmental triggers, such as medications, stress, substance abuse, sleep disorders, and changes of seasons. Treatment includes medications (mood stabilizers, anticonvulsants, and atypical antipsychotics). Antidepressants are contraindicated. Treatment with 1 drug (mood stabilizer) is the goal for older adults because of the potential for adverse effects and drug interactions because of co-morbidities. Electroshock treatment is effective for older adults with depressive states. The half-life of drugs, such as lithium, increases because of reduced renal clearance, so lower doses and careful monitoring are often necessary.

OCD

Obsessive-compulsive disorder (OCD) is a disorder in which patients are plagued by obsessions and/or compulsions that interfere with employment and social, interpersonal, and other daily activities and last more than 1 hour daily. Characteristics include:

- Obsessions are unwanted, repeated, and uncontrollable involving ideas, images, or urges that come to mind involuntarily despite attempts to ignore or suppress them.
- Compulsions are repeated, unwanted pattern(s) of behavior (impulses) to perform apparently irrational or useless acts that are often responses to obsessions and done to reduce stress. Examples include:
  o Cleaning and washing repeatedly to remove perceived contamination.
  o Repeated checking or counting.
  o Arranging and rearranging items.

A sense of dread may develop if the compulsion is resisted, and some try to ignore or suppress thoughts/behaviors. Intervention usually is not sought until emotional and/or physical exhaustion occurs in either client or a significant other. Differential diagnoses include depressive disorders, hypochondriasis, generalized anxiety disorder (GAD), Tourette's (may be a co-morbid condition), temporal lobe epilepsy, and schizophrenia.

Somatization disorder

Somatization disorder is characterized by physical symptoms not explainable by any known pathophysiological disorder but for which there is presumed to be a psychological basis. Common symptoms include nausea, vomiting, headaches, fatigue, and chronic pain. Indications include:
- Symptoms fulfilling a need to deal with a conflict.
- Symptoms not under voluntary control.

Somatization disorder occurs in females more than males and a familial tendency exists. Differential diagnoses include affective disorder, anxiety disorder, schizophrenia, depression, psychosis, hypochondriasis, and malingering. Mental status variations include:
- La belle indifference: An inappropriate relaxed attitude toward medical problems.
- Exceptional dependence.
- Appearing blind but not bumping into objects while walking.
- General dissatisfaction with the medical care received.
- Unawareness of relationship between psychological conflict and appearance of symptoms.

Depression in older adults

Depression affects about 19% of adults >55 and 37% of older adults with co-morbid conditions, putting older adults (who have the highest rates of suicide) at risk. Depression is associated with conditions that decrease quality of life, such as heart disease, neuromuscular diseases, arthritis, cancer, diabetes, Huntington's disease, stroke, and diabetes. Some drugs may also precipitate depression: diuretics, Parkinson's drugs, estrogen, corticosteroids, cimetidine, hydralazine, propanolol, digitalis, and indomethacin. Patients experience changes in mood, sadness, loss of interest in usual activities, increased fatigue, changes in appetite, fluctuations in weight, anxiety, and sleep disturbance. Depression often goes undiagnosed, so screening for at-risk individuals should be done routinely. *Treatment* includes tricyclic antidepressants (TCAs) and selective serotonin reuptake inhibitors (SSRIs), but SSRIs have fewer side effects and are less likely to cause death with an overdose. Older adults may take longer to respond to medication than younger adults. Counselling, treating underlying cause, and instituting an exercise program may help reduce depression.

Somatoform pain disorder

Somatoform pain disorder is characterized by chronic and constant pain for which there is no organic basis. Types include: acute (< 6 months) and chronic (> 6 months). Indications include:
- Symptoms may occur after physical trauma.
- Manifestations vary depending on the site of trauma.
- Patient develops fixation with pain.
- Pain is not relieved with analgesia.
- Patient may refuse to consider psychological origins.
- Depression is usually present.

Differential diagnoses include organic causes of pain, depression, anxiety disorder, hypochondriasis, conversion disorder, and malingering. Mental status variations include:
- Appearance: May assume a posture that minimizes pain.
- Behavior: Restless and appears uncomfortable.
- Mood: Depressed or apprehensive.
- Thought: Focused on pain.
- Concentration: Distracted or preoccupied.
- Insight: May be unaware or refuse to consider psychological factors.

Hypochondriasis

Hypochondriasis is the preoccupation with and fear of serious illness that lasts for 6 months despite medical reassurance that no physical pathology is present. Symptomatology may be related to an organ system, bodily function, or to a body part. Indications on the part of the patient include:
- Obsessed with personal health despite medical reassurance.
- May be able to admit that the fears are unrealistic.
- May recognize himself as a "hypochondriac" or may not recognize that concerns are exaggerated.
- May deal with fears by seeking information about diseases on the Internet, in books, or through other sources or may avoid the subject altogether.
- Tends to visit multiple clinicians.

Differential diagnoses include schizophrenia and the following disorders: generalized anxiety, body dysmorphic panic, delusional, conversion, and somatization.

Anorexia nervosa

Anorexia nervosa is an eating disorder characterized by:
- Refusal to maintain a minimal normal body weight.
- Extreme fear of becoming fat.
- Disturbed perception of body weight or shape.
- Denial of low body weight and high priority placed on weight or body shape in regards to self-evaluation.
- Amenorrhea for at least 3 consecutive menstrual cycles.

Anorexia nervosa may be restrictive without binging and purging or may include binging and purging. Anorexia nervosa is usually chronic and requires a lifetime of monitoring. Patients with anorexia nervosa exhibit many mental health symptoms and commonly have comorbidity with depression and dysthymia. They may be irritable, have sleep disturbances, experience lack of interest in sex, and withdraw from social interactions. They will be obsessed with the thought of food and may also have other obsessive-compulsive tendencies that may or may not involve food. They are at high risk for suicide. Characteristic physical findings (emaciation, amenorrhea, osteoporosis, hair loss, cardiac dysfunction) result from malnutrition and starvation.

<u>Laboratory findings</u>
Many of the abnormal lab findings with anorexia nervosa are associated with malnutrition and starvation. Some of the common lab findings include:
- Blood tests show decreased hemoglobin (anemia), leucopenia (depressed immune system), elevated blood urea nitrogen (BUN) (dehydration), high cholesterol, hypoglycemia (inadequate nutrition), elevated liver function studies, thrombocytopenia (decreased clotting ability), electrolyte imbalances particularly hypokalemia (low potassium), metabolic alkalosis or acidosis.
- Hormone levels show hypothyroidism and/or decreased estrogen, luteinizing hormone (LH), and follicle-stimulating hormone (FSH) levels.
- Electrocardiogram (ECG) may indicate dysrhythmias.
- Bone density tests show demineralization of bones and early-onset osteoporosis.

In the more severe cases, the patient can develop metabolic encephalopathy or increased ventricular/brain ratio, resulting from the complications of starvation. Anorexia nervosa can result in death.

Bulimia nervosa

There are 2 different types of bulimia nervosa:
- Restrictive: Similar symptoms to anorexia; however, after restricting eating for a period of time, patients will then binge eat and purge. This will become a cycle of behavior. Patients frequently fast, exercise excessively, and may or may not use laxatives and diuretics.
- Purging: Frequently utilize self-induced vomiting, laxatives, or diuretics in compensation for binge eating.

Many patients seeking treatment have co-morbid psychiatric disorders, including major depression, dysthymia, anxiety disorders, substance abuse problems, obsessive-compulsive disorder, post-traumatic stress disorder, personality disorders, and mood disorders. Criteria include:
- Repetitive cycles of binge eating.
- Use of inappropriate behaviors to prevent weight gain, such as induced vomiting; overuse of laxatives, diuretics or enemas; excessive exercise; or fasting.
- Binge eating along with inappropriate behaviors to prevent weight gain at least 2 times a week for at least 3 months.
- Patients influenced by body weight and shape when describing self.

<u>Physical, emotional, and laboratory findings</u>
Many of the physical and laboratory findings associated with bulimia nervosa are due to poor nutrition and self-induced vomiting habits. Physical symptoms can include loss of dental enamel or increased dental caries, chipped teeth, mouth sores, scars on dorsum of hand, cardiac and skeletal muscle myopathies, esophageal tears with associated bleeding, amenorrhea or irregular menstrual cycles, and decreased normal gastrointestinal functioning due to overuse of laxatives, often resulting in cycles of constipation and fecal impaction. Patients may engage in constant dieting and

exercise, exhibit signs of depression, hoard food, and have a distorted self-body image. Some of the associated laboratory findings result from repeated self-induced vomiting and laxative use and include fluid and electrolyte imbalances with increased blood urea nitrogen (BUN) and hypokalemia, metabolic alkalosis or acidosis, and elevated amylase levels.

Personality disorders

- Paranoid personality disorder: Characterized by extreme distrust and suspiciousness of others, assuming others have sinister motives.
- Schizoid personality disorder: Characterized as seeming indifferent to the praise or criticism of others, neither desiring nor enjoying close relationships.
- Schizotypal personality disorder: Exhibit very odd or strange behavior, associated with suspiciousness or paranoid ideation.
- Histrionic personality disorder: Excessive attention seeking and emotionalism associated with dramatic and seductive behavior and an unwarranted need for approval. It may be associated with concurrent somatization disorder in an effort to attract attention.
- Dependent personality disorder: Characterized by an over-reliance on others, submissive and clinging behavior, subordination of personal needs to those of others, and fear of separation. Patients often arrange for others to assume responsibility for the main areas of their lives. Patients lack self-confidence and may experience intense discomfort when alone for more than brief periods, feeling unable to cope without the help of others. This diagnosis should not be used when dependent behavior may be developmentally appropriate, such as in children and young teenagers.
- Passive-aggressive personality disorder: Characterized as passively complying with the desires of others while actually resisting complying. This condition manifests itself with resentment, claiming forgetfulness, procrastination, sullenness, or repeated failure to accomplish requested tasks for which one is responsible.
- Narcissistic personality disorder: Characterized by heightened feeling of self-importance, persistent patterns of grandiosity, a need for admiration, disregard for other people's rights, restraint in expression of feelings, and a lack of empathy.
- Obsessive-compulsive personality disorder: Characterized by a chronic preoccupation with rules, orderliness, control, emotional constriction, perseverance, stubbornness, and indecisiveness. Affection is usually expressed in a highly controlled fashion. This patient may be very uncomfortable in the presence of others who are emotionally expressive.
- Avoidant personality disorder: Characterized by extreme sensitivity to rejection that leads to feelings of inadequacy, mistrust of others, social withdrawal, and social inhibition. Patients often consider themselves socially clumsy, have exaggerated negative beliefs about themselves, and avoid social situations for fear of being ridiculed. This behavior is due to extreme shyness rather than a desire to be antisocial and should not be confused with shyness that is appropriate (such as from being a new immigrant).

BPD

The main feature of borderline personality disorder (BPD) is a persistent pattern of instability in interpersonal relationships, self-image, and emotion. Two-thirds of those diagnosed are female. Criteria include:
- Attempts to avoid real or imagined abandonment.
- Impulsivity in at least 2 of the following areas:
  o Spending.

- o Sex.
- o Substance abuse.
- o Reckless driving.
- o Binge eating.
- Recurrent suicide gestures.
- Self-mutilating behavior.
- Anger and rage outbursts.
- Unstable relationships.
- Identity confusion.

People with BPD feel insecure and inherently worthless. They are often erratic and have difficulty establishing long-term relationships, although symptoms tend to lessen with age. Theories about the causes of BPD include changing and unpredictable manners of parenting, genetic predisposition, emotional deprivation as a child, and/or sexual or physical child abuse.

Sexual dysfunctions

Sexual dysfunctions include:
- Male erectile disorder: Persistent or recurrent inability to achieve an erection and/or dissatisfaction with the size, rigidity, and/or duration of erections.
- Female sexual arousal disorder: Decreased, insufficient or absent ability to attain or maintain an adequate lubrication-swelling response to sexual excitement until the completion of sexual activity.
- Dyspareunia: Pain before, during, and/or after sexual intercourse.
- Vaginismus: recurrent or persistent involuntary spasm of the vagina, causing burning, pain and/or penetration problems.
- Orgasmic disorder: Persistent or recurrent delay in, or total absence of, orgasm associated with normal sexual activity.
- Premature ejaculation: Lack of voluntary control over ejaculation.
- Hypoactive sexual desire disorder (sexual anhedonia): Lack of sexual fantasies or desire for sexual activity.
- Sexual aversion disorder: Persistent or recurrent disgust, revulsion to, and avoidance of genital sexual contact with a sexual partner.

Primary insomnia, hypersomnia, and narcolepsy

Primary insomnia is difficulty falling asleep, staying asleep, a combination of both, and/or having non-refreshing sleep for at least 1 month, with onset usually after a stressful episode, resulting in impairment of work, study, and social activities. Patients may have anxiety and functional impairment and are at risk for mood disorders. Polysomnography may show that continuity of sleep is interrupted with increased alpha and beta waves during sleep although people usually are not sleepy in the daytime but may appear lethargic. They may also complain of stress-related disorders, such as muscle tension and headaches. Hypersomnia is characterized by increased sleepiness and prolonged sleep (8-12 hours or during the day on a daily basis for at least a month with difficulty awakening).
Narcolepsy is repeated periods of falling asleep during waking hours daily for at least 3 months. Narcolepsy can include catalepsy or recurrent rapid eye movement during the transition period between wakefulness and sleep, causing voluntary muscle paralysis and hallucinations.

Cannabis abuse

Cannabis abuse includes hashish, tetrahydrocannabinol (THC), and marijuana, also known as grass, dope, joint, weed, or J. Cannabis can be smoked or ingested. These drugs alter the user's state of awareness and can cause euphoria or dysphoria, sleepiness, heightened color and sound perceptions, red eyes, decreased inhibitions, dry mouth, increased appetite or tingling sensations. Overdose can lead to tachycardia, disorientation, or toxic psychosis. Disorders include:
- Dependence: Compulsive daily use for months or years, interfering with work, study, and social activities; sometimes associated with memory loss and general lethargy.
- Abuse: Periodic use that interferes with activities and social/family relations.
- Intoxication: Begins with "high" and includes inappropriate behavior/responses, memory impairment, sedation, difficulty acting, and sensory distortion. Severe anxiety, dysphoria, and perceptual disturbances (hallucinations) may occur.

There are usually no associated withdrawal symptoms; however, users can become irritable and may have insomnia for a few days.

Gender identity disorder

Gender identity disorder (gender dysphoria) exists when a male or female feels persistent discomfort with the gender of birth and a feeling that it is inappropriate or inaccurate. In children, criteria include 4 of the following:
- Repeatedly expresses a desire to be the other sex.
- In boys, a preference for cross-dressing; in girls, insistence on wearing only stereotypical masculine clothing.
- Believing that they will grow up to become the opposite sex.
- Having disgust with own genitalia.
- Using persistent references to opposite-sex roles in make believe play.
- Exhibiting intense desire to participate in the stereotypical games and pastimes of the other sex.
- Having a strong preference for playmates of the opposite sex.

In adolescents and adults, criteria include:
- A stated desire to live as a person of the opposite sex.
- Typically dressing as the opposite sex.
- Frequently passing as the opposite sex.
- A desire to be treated as the opposite sex.
- The conviction of having the feelings of the opposite sex.

Involuntary commitment of pediatric psychiatric patients

Involuntary commitment of pediatric psychiatric patients occurs in some instances. Assent is a productive and helpful aspect of treating pediatric patients. However, if the child does not assent, parents and guardians may still consent to therapy. Involuntary mental holds for 72 hours are sufficient to commence therapy. The legal premise behind these regulations is that parents act in good faith to ensure the wellbeing of their children. The legal guardian and healthcare provider are acting in place of the parents (*in loco parentis*). In most cases, the triage team on inpatient units has the option of deciding whether or not a patient should be admitted for evaluation or as protection for the patient's safety. For example, a teenager who attempts suicide may be placed on a 72-hour hold. Those healthcare professionals responsible for triage and treatment in the first 72 hours must act in the best interest of the patient and not under the influence of financial gain or parental desire.

Patient rights

Crucial psychiatric patient rights include:
- The right to informed consent: A patient is to be made aware of any procedure to be performed and must give permission on his or her own accord. Only court-ordered commitment procedures give hospitals the right to involuntarily treat patients.
- The right to refuse treatment: Patients may not be forcefully medicated; however, legal guardians can give permission if a court order is obtained. Patients may be forcibly medicated if they could possibly cause harm to self or others.
- The right to habeas corpus: Committed patients must be brought before a judge or court and must be released if insufficient reasons for confinement exist.
- The right to independent psychiatric examination: Patients may demand an evaluation by a mental health specialist of their choice and must be released if it is determined that they are not mentally ill.

Patient rights in psychiatric care

A right is a fair claim that is due to an individual, established by policies or laws. Important patient rights in psychiatric care include:
- Right to privacy: No information will be shared with unauthorized people about the patient. Exceptions include:
  o Presence of suspected child abuse.
  o Credible patient threats of physical harm to another. The potential victim must be alerted (per "Tarasoff" regulations).
  o During guardianship or involuntary commitment hearings.
- Right to treatment: Patients cannot be held against their will without an individualized treatment plan.
- Right to treatment in a least restrictive setting. Examples include:
  o Patients who pose no danger to themselves or others cannot be involuntarily hospitalized.
  o Patients who can function in an open ward cannot be held in a locked ward.
  o Clients who can live in the community and who have a support system must be treated in an outpatient setting.
  o Seclusion and restraint can only be utilized when it is in the patient's overriding best interest.

Patient interview

The patient interview is the first step in the process of treating a patient, and it is often where the most important information is obtained. Because it is such a crucial part of the overall assessment of the patient, it is important to make the patient feel comfortable. You are not likely to get a great deal of information from a patient if you make a negative impression. If possible, conduct the interview in a quiet area. If this is not a possibility, remain calm and relaxed as you interview the patient, and take your time both when asking questions and listening to the answers. If you give the patient the impression that you are impatient or in a rush, he or she may become uncomfortable and hesitant to answer questions.

Indifferent and permissive parenting

Parenting has an essential role in the social and behavioral development of the child. The degree of warmth the parents exhibit and the type of control have a profound effect on the child.

Style	Parental behavior	Effects on child
Indifferent	Shows little warmth and rarely imposes limits, may neglect or dislike child.	Child feels unloved and lacks direction or a positive sense of self, resulting in destructive or delinquent behavior.
Permissive	Shows much warmth and affection for the child but imposes few limits and little guidance although communication remains good.	Child may be creative and extroverted but doesn't negotiate or cooperate well with others, making acceptance by peers difficult. The child may become very self-centered and impulsive with impaired social functioning. The child may bully others or become aggressive and rebellious.
Authoritarian	Shows little warmth or affection for the child and communicates little. Is often inflexible and sets very restrictive limits that allow little independent thought or activity.	Child does not learn to negotiate or direct own behavior and has difficulty learning autonomy. Child may be fearful, passive, withdrawn. During adolescence, girls tend to be more passive and needy while boys tend to become aggressive.
Authoritative	Shows much warmth and affection for the child and provides guidance with minimal restraints. Maintains flexibility and communicates freely with the child, encouraging autonomy.	Child often has a positive self-image and is able to act independently and gets along well with others. The child is accepting of restrictions and often does well in school.

Differentiating delirium from depression, mania, and schizophrenia

Because delirium has symptoms in common with depression, mania, and schizophrenia, a careful history and physical examination may yield information to help differentiate among the disorders. The symptoms of delirium may have a sudden onset or may develop more slowly over a period of hours or days while the onset of symptoms of depression, mania, and schizophrenia usually have onset over a period of weeks to months. Delirium symptoms tend to be fluctuating while symptoms of the other disorders are more consistent. Additionally, delirium results from an underlying medical disorder, so if testing determines this disorder and the issue is resolved, then the symptoms generally abate. However, depression, mania, and schizophrenia, while they may occur with other disorders are not the result of those disorders. With depression, mania, and schizophrenia, patients' ability to conduct activities of daily living is often impaired, resulting in personal neglect of appearance; but this ability may or may not remain intact with delirium.

Mental health disorders due to renal and hepatic dysfunction

Renal/Uremic encephalopathy

This organic brain disorder results from increased toxins in the blood because of acute or chronic renal failure and a GFR of less than 15 mL/min. BUN and creatinine levels are markedly increased. Symptoms vary from fatigue to seizures and coma and may include confusion, impaired memory, emotional lability, somnolence, and asterixis (common) although the cause is unclear. Some medications, such as lithium and digoxin, may accumulate because of reduced renal function, contributing to encephalopathy. Treatment is dialysis, anemia reversal, and regulation of electrolytes.

Hepatic encephalopathy

This metabolic brain disorder is most often associated with cirrhosis of the liver and acute liver failure and results from increased levels of ammonia, which impair function of neurotransmitters and cause damage to astrocytes, inducing swelling of the astrocytes and cerebral edema. Symptoms are progressive, usually beginning with confusion and lethargy. Patients become increasingly somnolent and disoriented and then stuporous and finally comatose with decerebrate posturing. Motor activity decreases as the disease progresses, and asterixis is usually present. Treatment focuses on reducing hyperammonemia.

Mental health disorders associated with metabolic dysfunction

Severe mental health disorders, such as schizophrenia and mood disorders, are associated with metabolic dysfunction, referred to as the metabolic syndrome. This disorder is characterized by insulin resistance and glucose intolerance, obesity, high blood pressure, hyperlipidemia, and hyperuricemia. Patients with metabolic syndrome are at increased risk of diabetes mellitus and cardiovascular disease. Patients with severe mental illness often have high levels of cortisol as a reaction to stress, and this has been associated with increased visceral obesity, a contributing factor to diabetes and hypertension. Studies have shown that patients with schizophrenia tend to have increased rates of obesity, especially visceral obesity. Other studies indicate that those undergoing psychotic stress have impairment of beta-cell function in the pancreas and increased insulin sensitivity, and those with depression have increased risk of diabetes. Patients with bipolar also have increased rates of diabetes and high rates of obesity.

LBD

Lewy body dementia (LBD) is characterized by diffuse deposits of abnormal protein throughout the brain stem and other parts of the brain, including the cerebral cortex. Patients vary in symptoms but a primary feature is progressive dementia with decreased attention and impaired executive function. Cognition often fluctuates, and people typically experience visual hallucinations. Patients may experience falls, autonomic dysfunction, and other psychiatric abnormalities. Two features that are common to LBD and support the diagnosis are:
- REM sleep disorder: Patients act out their dreams physically, getting out of bed and carrying out activities. In some cases, patients may also talk or shout and may be physically violent, hitting or striking people or things. Treatment includes melatonin and/or clonazepam.

- Neuroleptic sensitivity: Up to half of the patients with LBD have severe sensitivity to neuroleptic/antipsychotic drugs and may develop increased cognitive impairment, severe sedation, increased or irreversible tremors/ Parkinsonism, and neuroleptic malignant syndrome, which may result in death. Antipsychotic drugs should be avoided with suspected LBD.

MMSE and Mini-Cog

Patients with evidence of dementia or short-term memory loss, often associated with Alzheimer's disease, should have cognition assessed. The Mini-mental state exam (MMSE) or the Mini-cog test is commonly used. Both require the patient to carry out specified tasks.
MMSE:
- Remembering and later repeating the names of 3 common objects.
- Counting backward from 100 by 7s or spelling "world" backward.
- Naming items as the examiner points to them.
- Providing the location of the examiner's office, including city, state, and street address.
- Repeating common phrases.
- Copying a picture of interlocking shapes.
- Following simple 3-part instructions, such a picking up a piece of paper, folding it in half, and placing it on the floor.

A score of ≥24/30 is considered a normal functioning level.
Mini-cog:
- Remembering and later repeating the names of 3 common objects.
- Drawing the face of a clock with all 12 numbers and the hands indicating the time specified by the examiner.

Health Promotion and Disease Prevention concepts

Screening tests must be designed according to a number of standards to ensure accuracy in results. Concepts include:
- Specificity: The ability to rule-out participants that should be excluded from further testing and do not have the diagnosis for which the screen tests.
- Sensitivity: The ability to accurately identify those who meet the criteria established by the test, providing diagnosis of a condition.
- Reliability: The ability to achieve similar results from repeated testing. Thus, if a condition remains unchanged, the test should provide similar results if given at a different time.
- Validity: The ability to achieve accuracy in results. Concurrent validity is supported by assessment within 10 days while predictive validity is supported by outcomes observed about a year after initial testing. Validity directly relates to both specificity and sensitivity.

AIMS

The Abnormal Involuntary Movement Scale (AIMS) is a tool to evaluate tardive dyskinesia in those taking antipsychotic medications. Before or after the exam, the patient is observed at rest (as in the waiting area) for comparison. The examination procedures include having the patient do a number of activities, such as sitting in specific positions, opening mouth, protruding tongue, standing, and walking while the nurse rates a number of characteristics on a scale of 0 (none) to 4 (severe):

- Facial and oral movements.
- Extremity movements.
- Trunk movements.
- Overall severity of movements.

These are assessed, and a score of ≥2 in 2 or more movement or a score ≥3 in 1 movement is positive. Then, the overall severity is assessed (based on the above scores), including patient's incapacitation, and patient's awareness of abnormal movements. The last part of the exam asks about dental status (problems, dentures, etc.).

CAGE

The CAGE acronym is used as a quick assessment tool to determine if people are drinking excessively or are problem drinkers. Moderate drinking, (1-2 drinks daily or 1 drink a day for older adults), unless contraindicated by health concerns, is usually not harmful to people, but drinking more than that can lead to serious psychosocial and physical problems. One drink is defined as 12 ounces of beer/wine cooler, 5 ounces of wine, or 1.5 ounces of liquor.

C	Cutting down	Do you think about trying to cut down on drinking?
A	Annoyed at criticism	Are people starting to criticize your drinking?
G	Guilty feeling	Do you feel guilty or try to hide your drinking?
E	Eye opener	Do you increasingly need a drink earlier in the day?

"Yes" on 1 question suggests the possibility of a drinking problem while "yes" on ≥2 indicates a drinking problem, and the patient should be provided information about reducing drinking and appropriate referrals made.

Confusion Assessment Method

The Confusion Assessment Method is used to assess the development of delirium and is intended for those without psychiatric training. The tool covers 9 factors. Some factors have a range of possibilities and others are rated only as to whether the characteristic is present, not present, uncertain, or not applicable. The tool provides room to describe abnormal behavior. Factors indicative of delirium include:

- Onset: Acute change in mental status.
- Attention: Inattentive, stable, or fluctuating.
- Thinking: Disorganized, rambling conversation, switching topics, or illogical.
- Level of consciousness: Altered, ranging from alert to coma.
- Orientation: Disoriented (person, place, time).
- Memory: Impaired.
- Perceptual disturbances: Hallucinations, illusions.
- Psychomotor abnormalities: Agitation (tapping, picking, moving) or retardation (staring, not moving).
- Sleep-wake cycle: Awake at night and sleepy in the daytime.

The tool indicates delirium if there is an acute onset with fluctuating inattention and disorganized thinking or altered level of consciousness.

Geriatric Depression Scale

The Geriatric Depression Scale is a self-assessment tool to identify older adults with depression. The test can be used with those with normal cognition and those with mild to moderate impairment. The test poses 15 questions to which patients answer "yes" or "no." A score of >5 "yes" answers is indicative of depression:
1. Are you basically satisfied with your life?
2. Have you dropped many of your activities and interests?
3. Do you feel your life is empty?
4. Do you often get bored?
5. Are you in good spirits most of the time?
6. Are you afraid that something bad is going to happen to you?
7. Do you feel happy most of the time?
8. Do you often feel helpless?
9. Do you prefer to stay at home rather than going out and doing new things?
10. Do you feel you have more problems with memory than most?
11. Do you think it is wonderful to be alive now?
12. Do you feel pretty worthless the way you are now?
13. Do you feel full of energy?
14. Do you feel that your situation is hopeless?
15. Do you think that most people are better off than you are?

Trail Making Test

The Trail Making Test (Parts A and B) assesses brain function and indicates increasing dementia. It is useful for detecting early Alzheimer's disease, and those who do poorly on part B often need assistance with activities of daily living (ADLs). The patient is given a demonstration of each part before beginning:
- Part A has 25 sequentially-numbered scattered circles across the page, and the patient is advised to use a pencil/pen to draw a continuous line to connect in ascending order the circles (starting with 1 and ending with 25).
- Part B is slightly more complex and has circles with numbers (1 to 12) and circles with letters (A to L) scattered about the page. The patient is advised to draw a continuous line alternating between numbers and letters in ascending order (1-A-2-B....).

The test is scored according to the number of seconds required for completion:
- A: 29 seconds is average, and >78 indicates deficiency.
- B: 75 seconds is average and >273 seconds indicates deficiency.

Digit Repetition Test and Time and Change Test

The Digit Repetition Test is used to assess attention. The patient is told to listen to numbers and then repeat them. The nurse practitioner starts with 2 random single-digit numbers. If the patient gets this sequence correct, the nurse then states 3 numbers and continues to add 1 number each time until the patient is unable to repeat the numbers correctly. People with normal intelligence (without retardation or expressive aphasia) can usually repeat 5 to 7 numbers, so scores ≤ 5

- 146 -

indicate impaired attention. The Time and Change Test assesses dementia in adults and is effective in diverse populations. Patients are shown a clock face set at 11:10 and have 1 minute to make 2 attempts at stating the correct time. The patient is then given change (7 dimes, 7 nickels, and 3 quarters) and asked to give the nurse $1.00 from the coins. The patient has 2 minutes and 2 tries to make the correct change. Failing either or both tests is indicative of dementia.

CGI scale

Clinicians use the Clinical Global Impressions (CGI) scale to compare ratings between patients he/she has already seen, usually for research studies. The CGI scale asks the clinician to rate the severity of illness on a scale of 0-7, in comparison to his/her "total clinical experience." Zero corresponds to "not assessed." Seven corresponds to "among the most extremely ill patients." The scale allows the clinician to rate the change or improvement seen after commencing a study drug. Additionally, an efficacy section of the CGI scale asks the practitioner to rate the therapeutic effects of drug treatments. The National Institutes of Health released a more consistent, revised scale in 1997 for bipolar disorder to allow clinicians to separate out side effects of drug treatment from actual improvement.

GAF scale

The Global Assessment of Functioning (GAF) Scale, developed for the Diagnostic and Statistical Manual of Mental Disorders (DSM), is a rating scale broken into 10-point subsections. Each 10-point GAF subsection has a corresponding description used by mental health practitioners to rate an individual's level of functioning. The highest score, 100, corresponds with "Superior functioning in a wide range of activities, life's problems never seem to get out of hand, is sought out by others because of his or her many positive qualities. No symptoms." The lowest score, 1, corresponds with "Persistent danger of severely hurting self or others (e.g., recurrent violence) OR persistent inability to maintain minimal personal hygiene OR serious suicidal act with clear expectation of death." A 0 (zero) score indicates there was inadequate information on which to base a rating

BPRS-C

The Brief Psychiatric Rating Scale for Children (BPRS-C) is designed to identify presenting symptoms and annotate the severity of each symptom, on a scale ranging from "not present" to "extremely severe." BPRS-C is used to diagnose psychiatric disorders for both children and adolescents through an interview with the child and parent(s). Symptoms evaluated on the scale include behavioral symptoms, such as uncooperativeness and hostility; mood symptoms, such as depressive mood and anxiety; sensory symptoms, such as hallucinations, delusions, and speech characteristics; symptoms of awareness and alertness, such as disorientation, hyperactivity, distractibility, and others; and symptoms of affect, such as emotional withdrawal and blunted affect. The BPRS-C assessment tool is a cursory look at many symptoms typically displayed with mental disorders.

Global Assessment Children's Scale

The Global Assessment Children's Scale is an adaptation of the Adult Global Assessment Scale (an earlier version of the Global Assessment Functioning Scale) from Axis V of the Diagnostic and Statistical Manual of Mental Disorders (DSM). This scale is applicable to children aged 4 to 16 years.

The categories of the scale include:

1-10	Needs constant supervision.
11-20	Needs considerable supervision.
21-30	Unable to function in almost all areas.
31-40	Major impairment in functioning in several areas and unable to function in a specific area.
41-50	Moderate degree of interference in functioning in most social area or severe impairment of functioning in 1 area.
51-60	Variable functioning with sporadic difficulties or symptoms in several but not all social areas.
61-70	Some difficulty in a single area, but generally functioning pretty well.
71-80	No more than slight impairment in functioning.
81-90	Good functioning in all areas.
91-100	Superior functioning.

CDRS-R

The Children's Depression Rating Scale-Revised (CDRS-R) evaluates a child for depressive disorders and monitors treatment response. CDRS-R includes 17 items, 14 of which are assessed during an interview, and 3 of which are assessed by the clinician's interpretation of the patient's non-verbal cues. The CDRS-R is designed specifically for patients aged 6 through 12 but may also be used during an interview with the patient's parents, caregivers, and teachers. The items included in the interview include the following: schoolwork; capacity to have fun; social withdrawal; sleep; appetite or eating patterns; excessive fatigue; physical complaints; irritability; guilt; self-esteem; depressed feelings; morbid ideation; suicidal ideation; weeping; depressed affect; tempo of speech; and hypoactivity.

SNAP-IV-C Teacher and Parent Rating Scale

The SNAP-IV-C Teacher and Parent Rating Scale is the revised version of the 1983 questionnaire by Swanson, Nolan, and Pelham. Clinicians ask parents and teachers to use SNAP-IV-C when attention-deficit/hyperactivity disorder (ADHD) or oppositional defiant disorder (ODD) is suspected. SNAP-IV-C allows parents and teachers to assess the child's propensity for moods and behaviors on a scale ranging from "not at all" to "very much." SNAP-IV-C includes 90 questions, which may help the clinician arrive at a diagnosis. Questions and topics include: the child's attentiveness; organization; physical and verbal activity; mood and temper (to include his/her ability to control the extremes of either); disruptiveness; attitudes towards authority, peers, and property; ability to concentrate; sleep patterns; self-esteem; anxiety; and ability to focus. Parent and teacher ratings tend to vary according to gender and poverty status; only teacher scores tend to vary by race.

HAS

The Hamilton Anxiety Scale (HAS or HAMA) is utilized to evaluate the anxiety-related symptomatology that may present in adults as well as children. HAS provides an evaluation of overall anxiety and its degree of severity. This includes somatic anxiety (physical complaints) and psychic anxiety (mental agitation and distress). This scale consists of 14 items based on anxiety-produced symptoms. Each item is ranked from 0 to 4 with zero having no symptoms present and 4 having severe symptoms present. This scale is frequently utilized in psychotropic drug evaluations. If performed before a particular medication has been started and then again at later visits, the HAS can be helpful in adjusting medication dosages based in part on the individual's score. It is often utilized as an outcome measure in clinical trials.

Y-BOCS

The Yale-Brown Obsessive Compulsive Scale (Y-BOCS) is a useful tool for identifying and diagnosing obsessive-compulsive disorders. Y-BOCS aims to identify obsessions, including: aggressive; contamination; sexual; hoarding/saving; religious; need for symmetry; somatic; and miscellaneous, such as cleaning/washing, checking, repeating, and counting. Y-BOCS asks the patient to rate the time he/she spends on obsessions and compulsions during the week prior to the clinician's interview. It asks the patient how much control he/she has over the compulsion/obsession, and how much distress it causes him/her. Y-BOCS has questions about resistance and interference. The clinician can ask for clarification and if the patient volunteers information, it is included in the assessment. The final rating is based on the clinician's judgment.

Drug screening

A drug screen is used to determine use of illicit drugs. Testing varies according to the type of drug used, duration of use, and time of use. Different types of screens include:
- Serum: Most drugs can be detected within 24 hours and for up to 3-5 days, but this varies.
- Saliva: Similar to serum, drugs can usually be detected within 1 to 3 hours of use and for 2 or 3 days afterward.
- Perspiration: The person wears a special patch for up to 2 weeks to evaluate chronic drug use.
- Urine: Drugs show up in the urine in about 6 to 8 hours, but tests can be inaccurate if people dilute urine by drinking 1 to 2 liters of fluids or add adulterants that change the chemical makeup of the urine.
- Hair: Drugs and alcohol can usually be detected in hair within about 2 weeks of use and remain for about 90 days.

BDI

The Beck Depression Inventory (BDI) is a widely utilized, self-reported, multiple-choice questionnaire consisting of 21 items, which measures the degree of depression. This tool is designed for use in adults between the ages of 17 to 80 years. BDI evaluates physical symptoms, such as weight loss, loss of sleep, loss of interest in sex, and fatigue, along with attitudinal symptoms, such as irritability, guilt, and hopelessness. The items rank in 4 possible answer choices, based on an increasing severity of symptoms. The test is scored with the answers ranging in value from 0 to 3. The total score is the utilized to determine the degree of depression. The usual ranges include:
- 0-9 (no signs of depression).
- 10-18 (mild depression).
- 19-29 (moderate depression).
- 30-63 (severe depression).

Functional assessment

ADLs

Functional status relates to the ability of people, especially the elderly or impaired, to perform social roles free of limitations or disabilities. Assessment should include basic activities of daily living (ADLs):

- Toileting: The ability to adequately control urination and fecal evacuation, noting dysuria, constipation, diarrhea, the presence and degree of incontinence, as well as the use of protective materials.
- Mobility: The ability to transfer from bed to chair, to walk, to toilet, and to maintain balance, noting recent falls or the need for assistive devices.
- Hygiene: The ability to bathe, brush teeth, dress, and maintain basic standards of cleanliness both for the person and the environment.
- Mental status: Thinking, understanding, and memory because, by age 90, about 50% of people have some dementia.
- Nutrition: Basic dietary knowledge, the ability to prepare or obtain food, and adequate food and fluid intake.

Psychosocial and sensory

Functional status assessment concerns the ability to do self-care, self-maintenance, and engage in physical activities, but other factors may prevent those who should be able to function well from doing so:

- Psychological function: Assess anxiety, worry, grief, and depression. Those with depression may be at increased risk of physical disability or may neglect self-care.
- Social function: Assess support from family or friends, the need for a caregiver, financial resources, mistreatment or abuse, the ability to drive, and the presence of advance directives.
- Sensory function: Assess presence of cataracts, glaucoma, myopia, presbyopia, astigmatism, macular degeneration, or eye disorders that make it difficult for people to read medication labels or do self-care. The need for audio materials or enlarged print should be assessed. Hearing is evaluated in both ears for hearing deficits and high and low frequency hearing loss as well as waxy buildup in the ear canals.

Universal principles of diagnostic testing

First, it is important to remember that the positive and negative predictive values of a test are not absolute. For example, if you test a high-risk population for diabetes (say 180 out of 200 have the disease), and then you test a low-risk population (20 out of 200 have the disease), the sensitivity and specificity of the test will stay the same, but the predictive values will change. Also, a test that has less than 100% sensitivity and specificity is most useful for the patient with an equivocal or intermediate probability of disease, rather than a high-risk patient or a low-risk patient. One other important point to remember is that sensitivity and specificity are inversely related. If a diagnostic test is modified in order to increase its sensitivity, the specificity of the test will decrease, and vice versa.

CT scans

If head injury is suspected, then the non-contrast CT is most commonly used because it is non-invasive and can be done more quickly than MRI. CTs can identify mass lesions, such as brain tumors, and acute intracranial hematomas and can indicate the presence of a midline shift as well as hydrocephalus. Fractures and pneumoencephaly can be detected. Hyperdense biconvex areas next to the skull indicate extradural hematoma, and hypodense regions within that hematoma indicate that active bleeding is occurring. Subacute subdural hematomas appear isodense in relation to brain tissue and are hard to identify although chronic subdural hematomas appear hypodense. Subarachnoid hemorrhage is indicated by a hyperdense area within the subarachnoid space. Intraventricular hemorrhage appears hyperdense. Diffuse axonal injury is usually not evident on CT although multiple small focal hypo- or hyperdense lesions may be noted. With cerebral edema, definition of the subarachnoid and ventricular spaces is lost.

Diagnostic reasoning process

There are a number of models for the diagnostic reasoning process but all essentially involve developing a hypothesis and testing it to arrive at a diagnosis. When diagnosing, a healthcare provider first looks for recognizable patterns of symptoms or presentation to suggest a diagnosis. If the patient does not fit a pattern, then a list of possible hypotheses is developed along with consideration of probabilities:
- Data is gathered and clustered.
- Diagnostic studies and assessment help to narrow the choice of hypotheses. Decisions are made about the type and extent of testing, including the sensitivity and specificity of different tests and the value of invasive vs non-invasive testing.
- Hypotheses are evaluated, using the gathered data and probabilities, to prioritize differential diagnoses.
- Treatment, based on the probable diagnosis, is provided and evaluated for efficacy. If treatment fails to bring improvement, then further hypothesis testing is indicated.

Importance of data gathering to diagnostic reasoning

The gathering and recording of data are of utmost importance to the diagnostic evaluation process. The history and physical section of the patient chart contains a wealth of information (ideally), and should always be taken into consideration when developing a care plan for the patient. Because any number of clinicians can add information to the patient chart (and because all of these clinicians will be reading this information), it is important to record all information clearly and in an organized manner. This can be a daunting task when you consider all of the different sources of information, including the patient interview, family member interviews, previous charts, and lab results. By keeping this information clear and concise, you can minimize error, and you can be sure that the differential diagnosis is comprehensive.

Problems that may be encountered during data evaluation

The data that are available on the patient chart are an integral part of the patient's overall care plan. However, errors may be present in the records, and these errors may negatively influence clinical decision making; thus it is important to look at the information as a whole. Does it make sense? Make sure that the patient's verbal history agrees with what you see in his or her records. Also, remember that not every test result you see in the patient's chart is necessarily accurate. If a test result doesn't make sense in the clinical picture as a whole, consider why this might be. It could simply be an error (e.g., the wrong number was recorded, the blood was drawn incorrectly), or the patient may have a result that would be considered "abnormal," though for this particular patient it is not. For example, a marathon runner may have a resting heart rate of 40 bpm; while this is a bradycardic rate, it is not pathological, but rather a result of physical conditioning.

Positive predictive value and negative predictive value

Predictive values are of importance to the clinician because although sensitivity and specificity are used to evaluate the effectiveness of a diagnostic test, they are not particularly clinically relevant. Since a patient's disease state is more or less unknown at admission, these parameters are of no help. This is where the positive predictive value (PPV) and negative predictive value (NPV) of a test come in. If your patient tests positive for syphilis, what are the chances that the patient actually has syphilis? The chance that this result is correct is the PPV; this is calculated by dividing the number of true positive results by the number of total positive results (true and false positives). NPV, then, is the probability that a patient with a negative result really does not have syphilis. Dividing the number of true negatives by the number of total negatives will give you the NPV.

Sensitivity and specificity

Some degree of error is inherent in almost all diagnostic testing. When you order a diagnostic test for a patient, how confident should you be that the result will be accurate? The terms sensitivity and specificity are used to illustrate the accuracy of diagnostic tests. The sensitivity of a test refers to its ability to correctly identify patients who do have the disease. If a test is administered to 100 patients with diabetes, and all 100 patients test positive, the test is considered to have a sensitivity of 100%. If only 85 of those tested have a positive result, however, that means that the test has a false-negative rate of 15%, and a sensitivity of 85%. On the other hand, the specificity of a diagnostic test refers to its ability to identify patients who do not have the disease. If 100 nondiabetic patients are tested for diabetes, and 50 of them have a positive result, the test has a specificity of only 50%.

Differential diagnosis process

The differential diagnosis is an important tool that allows the clinician to familiarize him or herself with the patient's condition, understand the condition, create an effective treatment plan, and follow the progress of the patient. To start, thoroughly examine the patient's chart, making a list of all of the abnormal test results and laboratory values. Add to this list all of the patient's complaints. Once this list is complete, organize the test results, labs, and complaints by anatomic location or organ system. After breaking the list down by organ site, look for any relationships between symptoms and/or results. Create another list of those data that seem to be related, and list all of the diseases or conditions that explain the findings, eliminating any that do not fit.

Influential factors on clinical decision-making process

Although one would like to think that there isn't much variation in the clinical decision-making process, this simply is not true. The process, of course, will differ depending on the patient, the differential diagnosis, and the clinician. First, let's start with the clinician. The way that the clinician conducts the clinical decision-making process is influenced by the knowledge base of the clinician, as well as the level of his experience, the ability he possesses to think both critically and creatively, and the confidence that he has in his ability to make educated decisions. The acuity level of the patient is also a factor in the clinical decision-making process, as is the length of the differential. A time stressor is placed on the clinician when the condition of the patient is critical, and when there are more diseases that must be eliminated from the differential. An element of stress may also exist if the clinician has a high number of patients, especially if he has multiple high-acuity patients.

Formulating a psychiatric diagnosis

The purpose of formulating a psychiatric diagnosis is to develop a plan of care to meet the needs of the patient. Steps include:

- History: Include the presenting problem and any initiating factors. Explain how the symptoms are affecting the patient's life. Note any prior history of psychological/psychiatric disorders as well as any history of disorders that may be associated with mental disorders, such as lupus erythematosus.
- Mental status exam: Note important or significant findings.
- Physical exam: Note any abnormalities. Diagnostic tests as indicated to rule out non-psychiatric conditions.
- Differential diagnosis: List only those that are plausible and must be ruled out.
- Single diagnosis: Base diagnosis on best evidence. In some cases, two diagnoses may be determined.
- Etiology: Note significant factors related to the diagnosis.
- Management plan: Outline the recommended treatment options to meet somatic needs (medications), psychological needs (therapy), and social needs (family intervention, support, community programs).

Practice Test

Practice Questions

1. Which of the following is NOT true about the epidemiology and risk factors of violent behavior?
   a. More than 50% of people who commit criminal homicides and who engage in assaultive behavior have imbibed significant amounts of alcohol immediately beforehand.
   b. For aggression classified as homicide, battery, assault with a weapon, or rape, the frequency among males clearly exceeds that among females.
   c. Most adults with and without mental disorders who commit aggressive acts do so against people they do not know, that is, strangers.
   d. For domestic violence, in which one partner hurts another, the frequency among men and women is about equal.

2. Your client is a 14-year-old girl brought in by her parents for evaluation because of episodes of defiance over curfews and of staying out late with friends. Your initial approach to her situation is which of the following?
   a. You meet with the family and tell the parents that such separation-individuation behavior is healthy and normal.
   b. You meet with the girl alone and explain that her behavior is exposing her to many high-risk behaviors, including substance abuse, delinquency, unprotected sex, pregnancy, and sexually transmitted diseases.
   c. You arrange for a separate therapist for the girl, a separate therapist for the parents, and yourself as the family counselor.
   d. You assess the family situation, assess the level of communication in the family, and attempt to identify specific stressors or situations that could be aggravating a normal development stage in order to address them.

3. You are working in a substance-abuse treatment clinic where the clients are subject to random, mandatory drug screening as a part of their probation for substance abuse–related offenses. If your client has a negative urine test result, you can be confident that the client has not abused any of the following drugs in the past 2 to 3 days EXCEPT:
   a. Heroin
   b. Toluene
   c. Cocaine
   d. Marijuana

4. Your client is a 34-year-old Hispanic-American farm worker who was diagnosed last year with bipolar disorder and who has been prescribed lithium carbonate. He came to the United States from Nicaragua 18 months ago. You are meeting him for the first time, after he has had 4 hospitalizations for his disorder and during which his lithium levels ranged from "undetectable" to 2.1 mEq/liter. What is the first step that you would take to assess his "health literacy" concerning his disorder?
   a. Determine whether he speaks English well enough to understand explanations and directions in English or whether he needs a translator.
   b. Ask him whether he was given information on bipolar disorder during and after his hospitalizations.
   c. Ask him to describe in his own words what his illness is and what he must do to manage it.
   d. Find out how much formal schooling he has had.

5. Which of the following is true about the heredity of bipolar disorder?
   a. The risk of one identical (monozygotic) twin having bipolar I disorder if the other twin has it is 75%.
   b. First-degree relatives of someone with bipolar disorder have a risk of developing bipolar disorder that is 4 to 6 times that of the general population.
   c. The risk of one fraternal (dizygotic) twin having bipolar I disorder if the other twin has it is 25%.
   d. If unipolar depression and bipolar I disorder are considered, then a co-twin has an even higher risk of affective illness if the index twin has bipolar I disorder, namely 100% for monozygotic twins and 50% for dizygotic twins.

6. The pathophysiology of major depressive disorder includes which of the following biochemical abnormalities?
   a. Cortisol secretion following administration of 1 mg of dexamethasone will be suppressed after 12 hours in 75% of patients with clinical signs and symptoms sufficient to diagnose major depressive disorder.
   b. Secretion of TSH following administration of TRH is suppressed in a significant proportion of patients with major depressive disorder relative to normal subjects.
   c. CSF levels of 5HIAA are elevated in the majority of patients with major depressive disorder who commit suicide.
   d. MHPG (3-methoxy-4-hydroxyphenylglycol), a metabolite of norepinephrine, is lower in the urine of patients with delusional depression than in patients with nondelusional depression.

7. Which of the following is required for the diagnosis of major depressive disorder?
   a. At least 1 week of persistently depressed mood.
   b. Suicidal ideation.
   c. The symptoms cause clinically significant distress or impairment of function.
   d. At least 4 of the following symptoms (depressed mood, loss of pleasure or interest, appetite or weight change, sleep disturbance, psychomotor agitation or retardation, fatigue, worthlessness or guilt, decreased concentration, and suicidal ideation) are present during most of 2 weeks and represent a change from the preceding 2 weeks.

8. A 25-year-old woman is brought by her family to the emergency room after complaining of having seizures again. She had been evaluated fairly recently for this same complaint, according to the family, but no medication was prescribed. The patient states that she doesn't like the neurologist and doesn't want him involved. You suspect that she is having pseudoseizures with a psychogenic etiology. What clinical observations or symptoms would help to confirm this possibility?

   a. Her seizures involve bilateral tonic/clonic movements during which she remains conscious and verbal.

   b. The patient holds her breath and becomes slightly cyanotic during an observed seizure in the ER.

   c. She reports having the olfactory hallucination of burning rubber just before the seizures.

   d. The patient and the family report that she is sometimes incontinent during the seizures.

9. A family brings in an elderly grandmother who is 87 years of age and who has been living with them. They express concern that she needs nursing home level of care. The patient's primary care physician evaluated her independently from the family and did not find a level of impairment or risk adequate to justify admission. You are called in to consult on the situation. Which of the following should be prominent in your differential diagnosis?

   a. Munchausen syndrome by proxy

   b. Malingering

   c. Substance abuse

   d. "granny dumping"

10. Which one of the following Axis II disorders requires the presence of an Axis I disorder as a diagnostic criterion?

   a. Borderline Personality Disorder

   b. Obsessive Compulsive Personality Disorder

   c. Schizoid Personality Disorder

   d. Antisocial Personality Disorder

11. A 32-year-old woman with Borderline Personality Disorder sees you in your private practice for medication management every 2 weeks. When you responded to a phone message while on call, she obtained your cell phone number and now calls you up to 5 times a day for crises. You should:

   a. Change your cell phone number and make sure that you block your number when returning calls to her in the future.

   b. Arrange to terminate your services with her and refer her for more comprehensive treatment at a mental health clinic or group practice that has a DBT or other specialized approach to these patients.

   c. Set limits on her phone calls, telling her that she may only leave messages on your business phone line (no more than once a day) and that you will return her calls at your discretion.

   d. Tell her that your contract with her is for office visits every 2 weeks and that you will not speak with her in between appointments.

12. You have obtained a position as a psychiatric nurse at a maximum security corrections facility. Many of your clients—who are men incarcerated for serious, violent crimes—complain of anxiety or insomnia and frequently request medication for help with these symptoms. Your response is to:
    a. Counsel them about progressive relaxation techniques—a non-medical approach to their symptoms.
    b. Assume that they are attempting to manipulate you to obtain drugs that will give them some kind of "high."
    c. Prescribe low-dose benzodiazepine medications that will be dispensed by the nurse on duty on an as-needed basis.
    d. Prescribe SSRI medications, which have no abuse potential and may help with anxiety symptoms.

13. You receive a notice from the pharmacy management service of your patient's insurance plan that he has been obtaining benzodiazepine medication from three other practitioners besides yourself, violating your agreement with him that you would prescribe these medications only if you were the sole provider. You decide that you will terminate treatment with this individual. You are concerned that he may become abusive, violent, or threatening if confronted with this directly. Your best course of action is which of the following?
    a. Leave him a phone message telling him that you are canceling his next appointment, not refilling any more prescriptions for him, and terminating your services as his clinician.
    b. At your next appointment, have a security guard or policeman present as you discuss the notice with him, give him a chance to respond to it, state that you believe that he is abusing these medications and may be dependent on them or addicted to them, suggest in-patient detoxification and substance abuse treatment, and inform him that you have decided that you can no longer treat him and will cease to be available as his clinician after 1 month, which will give him time to find another practitioner.
    c. Send him a registered letter (return receipt requested), in which you inform him of your decision to terminate with him as his clinician, cancel his next appointment, and tell him that you will be available for emergencies only for the next month, during which time he can seek alternative sources of treatment.
    d. Speak with him directly by phone to discuss the notice and its implications, give him a chance to respond to it, inform him of your decision to terminate with him as his clinician, suggest possibilities for in-patient detoxification and substance abuse treatment, and offer to be available by phone only for emergencies for 1 month while he seeks alternative treatment. Document the conversation fully in the medical record.

14. A challenging patient of yours with a paranoid personality disorder has gone to an emergency room with some physical complaints. The emergency room physician notices from his medical record that you are his psychiatric nurse, but the patient refuses to grant permission for the ER doctor to speak with you. The ER doctor calls you nonetheless, citing the Health Insurance Portability and Accountability Act (HIPAA), which states that clinicians may share information about patients for clinical purposes, and requests that you "fill him in" on the patient. What is your best response?
   a. You ask whether there is a life-threatening emergency that makes such a request legitimate under the laws of your state. If there is not, reply that you are unable to tell him anything about the patient because of confidentiality.
   b. Even though the ER physician is correct, you appreciate that there is a good chance that your patient will find out about your conversation and that you will risk disrupting your therapeutic alliance, given his diagnosis.
   c. Because there will be nothing in writing and it's just between the 2 of you, you provide some information to the ER doctor that will be helpful in managing your patient while he is in the ER in an effort to optimize his medical care.
   d. You ask the physician to put the patient on the phone and attempt to convince the patient that he should give you permission to speak with the ER doctor.

15. Your patient is a 70-year-old recently widowed woman who complains of initial insomnia as she works through her bereavement and requests something from you to help her with sleep. The best option of the following medications is:
   a. Flurazepam
   b. Diazepam
   c. Temazepam
   d. Eszopiclone

16. In initiating and monitoring pharmacotherapy with lithium carbonate, which of the following should be performed or measured done every 6 to 12 months?
   a. Electrocardiogram (ECG)
   b. BUN and creatinine
   c. Serum parathyroid hormone (PTH) level
   d. Dermatology consultation for psoriasis

17. Of the commonly prescribed antipsychotic medications for treatment of schizophrenia, which pair of the following drugs are most likely (first member of pair) and least likely (second member of pair) to cause weight gain, increased appetite, and abnormal glucose metabolism?
   a. Olanzapine (Zyprexa) and aripiprazole (Abilify)
   b. Quetiapine (Seroquel) and clozapine (Clozaril)
   c. Risperidone (Risperdal) and paliperidone (Invega)
   d. Perphenazine (Trilafon) and chlorpromazine (Thorazine)

18. A 25-year-old man complains of progressive symptoms of recurrent and persistent thoughts about germs and contamination experienced as intrusive and upsetting as well as feeling driven to perform repetitive hand washing, which has left his skin very dry and chapped. In addition to prescribing a selective serotonin reuptake inhibitor antidepressant, you recommend referral to a practitioner that specializes in:
a. Psychoanalysis
b. Therapeutic massage
c. Cognitive-behavioral therapy
d. Interpersonal psychotherapy (IPT)

19. The ethics manual of the American Psychological Association explicitly requires informed consent for psychotherapy, whereas informed consent for psychiatrists practicing psychotherapy is implicitly required in The Principles of Medical Ethics With Annotations Especially Applicable to Psychiatry. The advantages of obtaining informed consent from a patient before embarking on a course of psychotherapy include all of the following EXCEPT:
a. Informed consent ensures that the patient has been informed about the risks and benefits of psychotherapy and about available alternative treatments, which increases the ability of patients to help themselves and feel empowered in decision-making.
b. Informed consent lessens the risk of regressive dependency by deemphasizing any tendency for the patient to see the therapist as "special" or uniquely empowered to help the patient, making the patient an equal partner in the undertaking.
c. Informed consent acknowledges the uncertainty of outcomes in psychotherapy, making both the patient and therapist partners in the task of obtaining a positive result and allowing the therapist to have a more realistic role in the treatment process.
d. Informed consent, by interposing a more formal and legally based discussion between the therapist and the patient, tempers the formation of the therapeutic alliance and injects an element of doubt or negative perspective into the patient's hope for benefit.

20. As the nurse-in-charge of an in-patient psychiatric unit, you are present when your staff must intervene to forcibly restrain a 35-year-old man recently admitted with mania who has assaulted his brother, who was visiting him. You make the decision to place the patient in physical restraints so that he can be medicated and prevented from injuring others or himself. What is true about situations of this type?
a. Clients in restraints must be assessed every 30 minutes for circulation, respiration, nutrition, hydration, and elimination.
b. As soon as possible, but no longer than 1 hour after the initiation of restraint or seclusion, a qualified staff member must notify the physician of the patient's condition and obtain a verbal or written order for the restraint or seclusion.
c. Orders for restraints or seclusion of adults must be reissued by a physician every 8 hours.
d. A physician must evaluate the patient while in restraints every 24 hours.

21. A 56-year-old man whose wife died 1 year ago and who was recently diagnosed with inoperable lung cancer is brought to your clinic by his 32-year-old son, who expresses concern about his father's depressed mood. You conclude from your assessment that he has signs and symptoms sufficient to qualify for a diagnosis of major depressive disorder: 10-lb. weight loss, anhedonia, anergy, and some self-neglect of hygiene and clothing. He is lucid and competent, adamantly insists that he is not suicidal, does not have guns at home, is not at risk of injuring himself, and refuses recommended psychiatric hospitalization. He accepts a prescription for an antidepressant and an appointment for the next week. Two days later he dies of a self-inflicted gunshot wound. The son files a lawsuit for failure to diagnose and treat. Which of the following is true?
    a. If he deliberately concealed suicidal ideation and intent while competent and able to cooperate in a psychiatric examination, there is no liability.
    b. He should have been committed involuntarily to a psychiatric hospital for his safety because he had many risk factors for suicide.
    c. The son should have been instructed to determine whether his father had any firearms in the house and, if so, to remove them.
    d. Because he had lost 10 lbs. and was disheveled, he should have been committed involuntarily because of his inability to care for himself by reason of mental illness.

22. Which of the following organizations is responsible for the evaluation of standards for institutional healthcare?
    a. The Centers for Disease Control and Prevention (CDC)
    b. The National Center for Health Statistics (NCHS)
    c. The Joint Commission
    d. The Agency for Healthcare Research and Quality (AHRQ)

23. The American Nurses' Association (ANA), in collaboration with the American Psychiatric Nurses Association (APNA) and the International Society of Psychiatric-Mental Health Nurses (ISPN), has outlined a set of standards of practice that includes the following components of the nursing process:
    a. Coordination of Care; Health Teaching and Health Promotion; Milieu Therapy; Pharmacological, Biological, and Integrative Therapies; Prescriptive Authority and Treatment; Psychotherapy; and Consultation
    b. General Information, Predisposing Factors, Precipitating Event, Client's Perception of the Stressor, Adaptation Responses, Summary of Initial Psychosocial/Physical Assessment including Knowledge Deficits, and Nursing Diagnoses
    c. Assessment, Diagnosis, Outcome Identification, Planning, Implementation, and Evaluation
    d. Subjective Data, Objective Data, Assessment, Plan, Intervention, and Evaluation

24. You are meeting in your office with a 24-year-old man and his mother. His working diagnosis is schizophrenia, but he has become very depressed and is almost mute. His therapist and his mother agree that he should be hospitalized, but the mother would like him to be at the university hospital psychiatric unit, which will not have a bed available until the next day. The local community hospital psychiatric unit has a bed available immediately. Although he mumbles "no" to questions about suicidality, you feel that he should be hospitalized immediately because he is psychotic and unpredictable. Your supervisor is unavailable for consultation. What is the safest course of action?
   a. Allow the mother to take him home until tomorrow because she has agreed to take responsibility for monitoring him.
   b. Explain that you have no choice but to hospitalize him immediately, given your assessment, and instruct the mother to take him to the community hospital for admission.
   c. Ask the patient and his mother to sit in the waiting area while you make arrangements and then call the police and the ambulance service, fill out an involuntary commitment form, and wait for the police to arrive.
   d. Outline your recommendation that the patient be admitted immediately. State that you will arrange for him to be taken to the community hospital by ambulance and that you will assist with the transfer to the university hospital psychiatric unit the next day, if possible. Explain that you would prefer to avoid an involuntary commitment action but that you are willing to do so if the family does not agree to the plan.

25. You have noticed that your clients who take a multivitamin daily seem to suffer less from upper respiratory infections and have less trouble with depression. You decide to perform a small study to determine whether the vitamin C and vitamin D content of the multivitamins is a factor. You obtain funding; obtain IRB approval; arrange for the preparation of identical capsules containing placebo, vitamin D, vitamin C, or both vitamins; and arrange for patients, as they come for their appointments, to be randomly assigned into the treatment groups. The contents of the capsules given to a particular patient will be unknown to you, the clinicians, and the patients. This type of clinical trial is called:
   a. A double-blind, placebo-controlled clinical trial
   b. A case-control study
   c. A single-blind, placebo-controlled clinical trial
   d. A cross-sectional study

26. Which of the following statements are true about risk of suicide?
   a. Suicide risk declines with age, reaching its lowest level among persons 65 years of age and older
   b. Of all racial groups, African Americans have the highest suicide risk
   c. Women have a higher risk of completed suicide per attempt than do men
   d. Suicide risk is elevated by a history of suicide in a first-degree relative, especially the same-sex parent

27. Motivational interviewing for reduction of high-risk behaviors includes which of the following components?
   a. Vigorous confrontation of resistance to change
   b. Maintenance of a detached, impersonal attitude
   c. Encouragement of the client to accept the therapist as authoritative and to foster dependency
   d. Developing discrepancy by helping the client to see how their day-to-day behavior deviates from their ideals

28. Which of the following situations does NOT correlate with an increased risk of vulnerability to unhealthy levels of stress?
    a. Working more than 48 hours per week
    b. Having been divorced or separated in the past year
    c. Having a network of friends and acquaintances
    d. Drinking alcohol, smoking, or using drugs to relax

29. All of the following are questions included in the CAGE screening test for alcohol problems EXCEPT:
    a. Have you ever felt you should cut down on your drinking?
    b. Have you ever annoyed people by your drinking?
    c. Have you ever felt bad or guilty about your drinking?
    d. Have you ever had a drink first thing in the morning to steady your nerves or to get rid of a hangover (eye opener)?

30. The following prevalence rates for schizophrenia in specific populations are accurate EXCEPT:
    a. General population   1%
    b. Non-twin sibling of a schizophrenic patient   16%
    c. Child with one schizophrenic parent   12%
    d. Child of two schizophrenic parents   40%

31. A 23-year-old man presents to the emergency room requesting referral for opiate detoxification and complaining of withdrawal symptoms. On physical examination, you find all of the following signs and symptoms EXCEPT:
    a. Rhinorrhea and lacrimation
    b. Constricted pupils (miosis)
    c. Profuse diarrhea
    d. Piloerection (gooseflesh)

32. A 17-year-old adolescent girl is brought to you by her parents, who complain that she doesn't eat and is very thin. On examination it is determined that her body weight is less than 85% of normal, she has not had a menstrual period in 6 months, she worries about being overweight, and she complains that she is "too fat." Which of the following additional features allows you to confidently diagnose Anorexia Nervosa, Binge-Eating/Purging Type as a single diagnosis rather than Bulimia Nervosa additionally?
    a. Binging and purging occur only during episodes of anorexia nervosa
    b. Episodes of binge eating are recurrent
    c. Inappropriate compensatory behavior to prevent weight gain—such as self-induced vomiting, use of diuretics or laxatives, fasting, or excessive exercise—is recurrent
    d. Binge eating and inappropriate compensatory behaviors have both been occurring, on average, at least twice per week for 3 months

33. Which of the following features supports the diagnosis of Malingering, as opposed to Factitious Disorder?
   a. Medical history, physical examination, and laboratory evaluations do not identify specific abnormalities
   b. The patient's symptoms have necessitated his being kept in the hospital rather than returning to prison to continue serving his sentence
   c. The patient's symptoms are vague, ill-defined, at times overdramatized, and not in accordance with known clinical conditions
   d. The patient has a long history of previous hospitalizations, during which his symptoms have been severe but little pathologic evidence has been identified

34. Which of the following is the most helpful in distinguishing a syndrome of Dementia from one of Delirium?
   a. The patient has a fluctuating level of consciousness
   b. The patient is disoriented to person, place, and time
   c. The patient is unable to remember more than 1 of 3 objects at 3 minutes
   d. The patient keeps asking of the whereabouts of his spouse, who died last year

35. You are conducting an assessment of a 37-year-old unmarried mother of 4 who works as a unit clerk at the local community hospital. In reviewing her level of functioning in various areas, which of the following stands out to you as needing attention and exploration?
   a. Her children attend school regularly, earn above-average marks, have friends, and receive positive reports from their teachers
   b. She is financially stable, making ends meet with her salary and with some help from extended family for occasional childcare needs
   c. She obtained restraining orders, through Legal Aid services, on two former boyfriends who became abusive and exploitative
   d. Despite having to take time away from work to help her youngest child get treatment for severe asthma, she negotiated with her employer to use vacation and sick time from the coming year and took minimal unpaid leave under the Family Medical Leave Act (FMLA)

36. Which of the following is a warning sign that a nurse is in danger of crossing the professional boundary of the nurse-client relationship?
   a. A married patient of the same sex, with whom you have worked for several years through several crises, brings you a small box of candy as a gift just before the Christmas holidays
   b. You find yourself anticipating appointments with an attractive single patient and paying special attention to how you dress and wonder whether the patient finds you attractive
   c. A patient who is a parent confides her distress over the serious illness of one of her children and you mention that one of your children had been similarly ill in the distant past and that you can understand somewhat what she must be going through
   d. A patient of the opposite sex, whom you have known for some time, has confided to you that his or her parent died unexpectedly the previous week and spends much of the session grieving and tearful. At the end of the session, the patient embraces you in appreciation and you reciprocate, holding the patient in your arms for a few seconds before the patient departs

37. A married Italian man in his 60s has a history of treatment-resistant depression. You consult with the patient's psychiatrist, and the recommendation is to initiate treatment with an MAO inhibitor antidepressant. What is the most important reason to meet with the patient's family when you prescribe this medication?
   a. MAO inhibitors can cause orthostatic hypotension, which may be worse on arising; therefore, family members need to be watchful
   b. MAO inhibitors can cause sexual dysfunction; therefore, the patient's spouse should be informed so as to anticipate this possibility
   c. MAO inhibitors can interact with certain foods and over-the-counter medications and cause an abrupt increase in blood pressure, which can be harmful
   d. MAO inhibitors can disrupt the sleep-wake cycle, which can result in daytime somnolence and nighttime insomnia

38. Evidence-based treatment approaches to Attention-Deficit Hyperactivity Disorder (ADHD) include all of the following EXCEPT:
   a. Progressive relaxation techniques and meditation
   b. Stimulant medication and monitoring of heart rate and blood pressure
   c. Behavioral parent training (BPT) and behavioral classroom management (BCM)
   d. Intensive peer-focused behavioral interventions implemented in recreational settings (e.g., summer programs)

39. All of the following medication interventions would be reasonable as a next step in the treatment of Major Depressive Disorder when the patient has only partially improved after 6 to 8 weeks in response to an adequate dose of a standard SSRI antidepressant (e.g., fluoxetine, sertraline, fluvoxamine, paroxetine, citalopram, or escitalopram) EXCEPT:
   a. A second SSRI
   b. The switch to an MAO inhibitor antidepressant
   c. A tricyclic antidepressant, such as nortriptyline or desipramine
   d. The addition of lithium carbonate

40. Which of the following is NOT an important reason for monitoring lithium therapy with periodic blood tests?
   a. Long-term use of lithium may be associated with a decline in renal function, as indicated by elevations in BUN and creatinine levels
   b. Lithium may exacerbate psoriasis
   c. Lithium has been associated with elevated levels of parathyroid hormone and hypercalcemia in some patients
   d. Lithium can cause elevations in thyrotropin (TSH) and subclinical or clinical hypothyroidism, much more frequently in females than in males

41. All of the following situations support the use of psychotherapy EXCEPT:
   a. The therapist maintains a neutral demeanor as a "blank canvas" to facilitate transference
   b. The objective of the therapist is to reinforce the patient's healthy and adaptive patterns of thought and behavior
   c. The therapist engages in a fully emotional, encouraging, and supportive relationship with the patient
   d. One aim of the treatment is to strengthen healthy defense mechanisms, especially in the context of interpersonal relationships

42. Which of the following statements is true concerning the use of phototherapy for Seasonal Affective Disorders?
   a. Light therapy must be used to extend the period of daylight artificially by exposure before sunrise or after sunset
   b. The optimum time of day for treatment is during the evening
   c. A session must last at least 2 hours for any positive effect to occur
   d. Evidence indicates that the wavelengths of light in the blue-green end of the visual spectrum are as effective as white light

43. Which of the following statements is NOT true about informed consent?
   a. Adult patients are assumed to have the right to consent to or refuse treatment
   b. Sufficient information about the diagnosis, the prognosis, and the risks and benefits of the proposed treatment must be provided
   c. The provider is not required to inform the patient of the risks and benefits of possible alternative treatments, including no treatment at all
   d. A procedure performed without informed consent is considered battery and may be malpractice as well

44. Nurses are mandated to report abuse or neglect in all of the following situations EXCEPT:
   a. A 12-year-old boy being seen for ADHD medication appears malnourished and has visible bruises on his forearms
   b. A 35-year-old woman complains that her boyfriend often forces her to have sex when she is unwilling and that she is distressed by this and unsure of what to do about it
   c. An 82-year-woman who lives with her son and daughter-in-law recounts that she doesn't know what happens to her Social Security check every month and that her family refuses to discuss it with her, telling her "it's taken care of"
   d. An 8-year-old girl tells you that she dislikes being left at her grandfather's house because he cajoles her into playing games during which they dress and undress in front of each other and then wrestle on the floor

45. A 42-year-old married man brought to the hospital by police is agitated, claims not to have slept for 3 days, believes that God has revealed a special mission to him to meet with the President of the United States and confront him directly about the budget deficit, and says he will pursue this or die trying. He was found wandering on the street in his underwear in mid-January in New England, and his wife states that he has not been eating. All of the following are reasons for which he may be involuntarily committed for psychiatric care by reason of mental illness EXCEPT:
   a. He presents a danger to others, specifically to the President of the United States
   b. He is a danger to himself because his behavior, if unchecked, would certainly cause security personnel to stop him from approaching the President of the United States, with deadly force if necessary
   c. His lack of sleep, being underdressed for the weather, and not eating suggest that he is unable to care for himself in his current state
   d. His wife reports that he has been spending money irresponsibly, risking financial ruin for the family

46. Which of the following is an example of 1 of the 4 stages of cognitive development identified by Piaget?
    a. Formal Operations (12-15+ years)
    b. Preconventional Level (ages 4-10 years)
    c. Toddlerhood (learning to delay satisfaction)
    d. The Symbiotic Phase (ages 1-5 months)

47. Which of the following is NOT considered Personal Health Information (PHI) under the Health Insurance Portability and Accountability Act (HIPAA)?
    a. Biometric identifiers, including finger and voice prints
    b. The name of the patient's attending physician
    c. Device identifiers and serial numbers
    d. Internet Protocol (IP) address numbers

48. The family of an elderly patient with a recent diagnosis of terminal cancer takes you aside and requests that you not inform the patient of the diagnosis because it would be too upsetting for them. You conduct an assessment and find that the patient is competent and rational. The patient asks you to discuss the doctor's findings, and you focus on the patient's mild chronic history of asthmatic bronchitis. Which ethical principle have you violated?
    a. Beneficence
    b. Justice
    c. Veracity
    d. Nonmaleficence

49. Which is the best reason for obtaining a consultation?
    a. The possibility exists that a diagnosis might be incorrect and obtaining a second opinion will provide greater protection from a lawsuit
    b. The patient's condition is complex and interesting, and you know that the consulting psychiatrist will consider the case of interest in teaching nurses and medical students
    c. Your supervisor has encouraged you to obtain consultations more frequently because you don't seem to ask for help often enough and he or she is concerned that you might be overlooking subtleties or ignoring complexities
    d. The patient's situation is complicated by many psychosocial and medical issues and you are not certain which course of treatment will be most advantageous; you believe that proper care demands additional expertise

50. The following are 4 of the criteria used to evaluate qualitative research. Which of them is incorrectly defined?

    a. Descriptive Vividness – The researcher describes the data gathering process in sufficient detail that the reader can personally experience it. The data collected, often in the form of personal statements, should be quoted directly and extensively, because this is the raw data from the study

    b. Methodological Congruence – The researcher presents the philosophical and methodological approach used and cites references to support their approach. The subjects, sampling method, data-gathering and data-analysis strategies, and processes for informed consent are clearly and concisely described

    c. Analytical Precision – The methods used to determine statistical significance, study size, the number of subjects needed, and the precision and accuracy of the instruments used to measure the data are described in detail

    d. Theoretical Connectedness – Any theory developed from the study is clearly stated, logically consistent, reflective of the data, and in accord with other available knowledge

Answers and Explanations

1. C: Most aggressive acts are committed against people who are known to the aggressor, usually family members. The exceptions to this general rule are male adolescents, who may act violently against acquaintances who they know only slightly or against complete strangers.

2. D: The important first step is a thorough assessment of the situation, i.e., asking lots of questions before making any suggestions. Subsequently, the practitioner can assess the client's level of education and vulnerability concerning high-risk behaviors, determine whether separate therapists are indicated, and determine the degree to which the behavior is normative or pathological.

3. B: Toluene is a constituent of solvents that are abused through inhalation. Like most of the substances abused through inhalation, toluene is not detected by urine drug screenings. Other means of assessing inhalant abuse, such as detecting the odor of the inhalant on the subject's breath (where it may persist for many hours) or finding products of abuse stored in unusual locations, must be sought.

4. A: Given this history, the patient is unlikely to have a strong grasp of the English language, adding an additional degree of difficulty to developing his "health literacy," that is, his "capacity to obtain, process, and understand basic health information and services needed to make appropriate health decisions." Being able to provide information and education in a language that he can understand is the first step, preceding even an assessment of his understanding.

5. B: The majority of studies show a concordance of 40% for monozygotic twins and 0 to 10% for dizygotic twins. When unipolar depression and bipolar I disorder are considered, the risk is 69% for identical twins and is 19% for fraternal twins when the index twin has bipolar I disorder.

6. B: The response of TSH to TRH is blunted in a significant proportion of patients with major depressive disorder. The dexamethasone suppression test is positive (that is, cortisol is not suppressed) in only about 50% of patients with major depressive disorder. CSF levels of the serotonin metabolite 5HIAA are significantly reduced in patients who commit suicide. MHPG is elevated in the urine of patients with delusional depression compared with patients without delusional depression.

7. C: Either depressed mood or loss of interest or pleasure must be present for 2 weeks. Suicidal ideation need not be present for the diagnosis, but at least 5 of the listed symptoms must be present for 2 weeks. There must be clinically significant distress or impairment of function caused by the symptoms.

8. A: Patients may remain conscious during unilateral, partial motor seizures; however, the spread of the seizures to both cerebral hemispheres (indicated by bilateral tonic/clonic movements) is always associated with loss of consciousness. The other symptoms are frequently seen during seizure disorders.

9. D: Munchausen by proxy (factitious disorder by proxy) usually involves a parent who presents a child repeatedly for treatment with physical complaints or conditions that turn out to be fabricated or produced by the parent, who is motivated by a wish to adopt a sick role vicariously through the child. Malingering would usually be manifest by the adoption of feigned or exaggerated symptoms in order to obtain nursing home admission, when the patient has minimal signs and symptoms. If

the patient has an occult substance abuse problem that causes serious impairment at home but not when sober, as here when seen by the physician, it could explain the disconnect. However, the family is usually aware of and reports the substance abuse. "Granny dumping," the attempt to offload a burdensome elder onto the healthcare system, must be considered prominently in the differential diagnosis, given the limited information.

10. D: Antisocial Personality Disorder requires evidence of a Conduct Disorder with onset before age 15 years.

11. B: Patients with this degree of behavioral dyscontrol should not be managed by a solo practitioner in a private office setting. You need to terminate your services and help her find an alternative venue that will more comprehensively manage her neediness and dilute her transference over a wider group of clinicians.

12. A: Many incarcerated individuals have antisocial personality disorders and will attempt to manipulate or con susceptible prison staff, often seeking drugs or diagnoses that will gain them special treatment. Malingering (making up symptoms to gain an advantage) is common in this population. Individuals feigning symptoms for this purpose will generally be uninterested in non-medical approaches, allowing some differentiation between a malingering population and those with a genuine problem.

13. D: You are not required to expose yourself to undue risk of injury or even abuse from a potentially violent patient. The compassionate and correct way to terminate your services is to speak with the patient directly, by telephone if an office visit will present too great a risk, and inform them of your decision and why you are making it, offering to help arrange additional treatment for substance abuse issues. Full documentation in the medical record and in a registered letter and the offer to be available on an emergency basis for 1 month will protect you against any accusation of abandonment. Offering to help arrange in-patient detoxification will protect you against any liability should the patient refuse and then have withdrawal complications.

14. A: If state confidentiality statutes are more restrictive than the federal guidelines of HIPAA, the former take precedence. Here, there has been no compelling reason presented to you that would supersede your explicit contract of confidentiality with the patient about his privileged information. Although the consequences of sharing information without his permission may be greater, given his paranoid personality disorder, that alone should not be the rationale for deciding to share confidential information or not. Also, attempting to speak with the patient if he has not requested it would generally be too involved or intrusive to be positive for the treatment alliance with this type of patient.

15. C: Both flurazepam and diazepam have long elimination half-lives and are not recommended for use in patients over the age of 65 years. Eszopiclone is likely to be more expensive than the other agents listed, which are available in generic form. Temazepam has an intermediate half-life, is FDA-approved for insomnia, and is well-tolerated and inexpensive.

16. B: Deterioration of kidney function with long-term lithium use is a significant risk, requiring BUN and creatinine to be monitored at least annually. Whereas lithium can cause T wave changes in the ECG and can exacerbate or precipitate psoriasis in some patients, there is no need to monitor these areas in any regular way. Lithium has been associated with elevations in serum parathyroid hormone and serum calcium, but not frequently enough to be routinely monitored.

17. A: The newer second-generation antipsychotic medications have demonstrated a tendency to significantly increase appetite, weight, and glucose intolerance. Clozapine and olanzapine are the most likely, risperidone and quetiapine are less likely, and ziprasidone (Geodon) and aripiprazole are least likely to be associated with these adverse effects.

18. C: Although Obsessive Compulsive Disorder is clearly an Axis I condition mediated by abnormalities in brain function and neurotransmitter balance, good empirical evidence indicates that the application of behavioral techniques such as exposure and response inhibition are effective in motivated patients for improving symptom control.

19. D: The hazard of psychotherapeutic informed consent is that it interferes with the establishment of initial rapport and therapeutic alliance by fostering discouragement and a negative suggestion about the possible outcome of the treatment. The other choices are the benefits of informed consent for psychotherapy.

20. B: Patients in restraints or seclusion must be observed and assessed every 10 to 15 minutes for circulation, respiration, nutrition, hydration, and elimination. Orders for restraints or seclusion must be reissued by a physician every 4 hours for adults (every 2 hours for those aged 9 to 17 years and every 1 hour for children younger than 9 years), and a physician must evaluate the patient while in restraints or seclusion every 8 hours (18 years and older) or every 4 hours (younger than 18 years). (The Joint Commission Guidelines)

21. A: In the absence of any stated or implied suicidal ideation or intent and without evidence of very significant self-neglect, involuntary hospitalization in this case would have been beyond the scope of the usual statutes governing such interventions, which usually require "likelihood of serious harm" or "substantial risk" of injury to self or others. If the patient is assessed as competent, the clinician cannot be held liable for the patient's deliberate withholding of suicidal ideation or intent and of information about possession of lethal means or for the patient's failure to seek help when such suicidal ideation or intention arose.

22. C: The CDC provides information for health protection and disease prevention, including environmental health and occupational health and safety and infectious disease monitoring. The NCHS compiles health statistics to guide policy formation in the health care field. The AHRQ develops clinical guidelines and promotes evidence-based medical practices. The Joint Commission performs periodic reviews of hospital care, including areas of operations, staff performance, physical facilities, and standard operating procedures. If the institution meets standards of practice in these areas, it is given initial or ongoing accreditation. The Joint Commission is a non-profit organization that has been accrediting institutions since 1951. Accreditation by the Joint Commission is often required by health insurance plans for coverage of services.

23. C: The elements of answer (a) are those of the Implementation component of nursing process. The elements of answer (b) are those of the Assessment component of the nursing process. The elements of answer (d) are those of the Documentation aspect of the nursing process.

24. D: Although family members might be willing to "take responsibility," they are not trained mental health professionals and you will be liable for any adverse outcome resulting from delaying the admission overnight. Even expecting the mother to follow through on taking her son to the community hospital is risky, because she could decide to drive him home instead. An involuntary commitment without discussion with the family would be needlessly challenging to the therapeutic alliance, unless your assessment is that the patient would run away if he knew that he would be

taken to the community hospital immediately, instead of waiting for a bed to become available at the university hospital. Sending the patient voluntarily by ambulance is the best route, if the family agrees, with involuntary commitment as the fallback option.

25. A: When both the subject and the investigator are "blind" to the treatment option being given, it is a "double-blind" trial. When only the subject is unaware of which treatment is being given, it is a "single blind" trial, which is considered to be subject to investigator bias because the latter knows the treatment being given and may be influenced to assess it as more effective in the subjects receiving it. Cross-sectional studies make observations in subjects at a single point in time, whereas a case-control study identifies subjects with the condition and compares them with a sample of subjects without the condition to determine which other factors are associated with the difference in outcomes.

26. D: Suicide risk increases with age and is highest in persons older than 65 years. Whites have the highest rate of suicide, followed by Native Americans, African Americans, Hispanic Americans, and Asian Americans. Women attempt suicide at a higher rate than do men, but men succeed more often.

27. D: Motivational interviewing is a client-centered approach that involves "rolling with the resistance" rather than confronting it, expressing empathy and viewing the situation from the client's perspective, supporting self-efficacy by explicitly embracing client autonomy, and developing discrepancy.

28. C: Some of the many factors that increase stress levels are social isolation, financial instability, job loss, divorce or separation, and physical illness. Signs of stress include irritability, loss of interest, sleep disturbance, weight loss, increased use of alcohol or drugs, increased use of sick time from work, and increased levels of physical complaints and symptoms.

29. C: The correct form of question "c" is "Have people annoyed you by criticizing your drinking?" The others are correct formats from the CAGE (Cut down, Annoyed, Guilty, Eye opener) assessment for alcohol problems.

30. B: The prevalence of schizophrenia among non-twin siblings of a schizophrenic patient is 8%. Being a dizygotic twin of a schizophrenic patient raises the prevalence rate to 12%, and being a monozygotic twin of a schizophrenic patient raises the prevalence rate to 47%.

31. B: Opioid Withdrawal Syndrome is associated with severe muscle cramps and bone aches, profuse diarrhea, abdominal cramps, rhinorrhea, lacrimation, piloerection or gooseflesh, yawning, fever, pupillary dilation (mydriasis), hypertension, tachycardia, and temperature dysregulation.

32. A: If a patient binges and purges only during periods of time when other signs and symptoms qualify the patient for a diagnosis of Anorexia Nervosa, Bulimia Nervosa will not be diagnosed additionally. The correct diagnosis in this situation is Anorexia Nervosa, Binge Eating-Purging Type.

33. B: In both Factitious Disorder and Malingering, false or grossly exaggerated physical or psychological symptoms are intentionally reported. Careful assessment both excludes other causes and often allows documentation of direct evidence of fabrication based on the non-physiological or non-anatomical nature of the symptoms, changes in symptoms, or observations (e.g., witnessing a patient deliberately contaminate a wound that mysteriously refuses to heal). There may be a pattern of such "illnesses" in both cases. Malingering is associated with a clear external incentive or

secondary gain from assuming a sick role, such as avoiding military service or incarceration, avoiding work, obtaining financial rewards such as disability payments or other financial compensation, obtaining drugs, or evading criminal prosecution. Factitious Disorder is associated with a more internal motive, that is, to assume the sick role.

34. A: Deficits in cognition can be similar in delirium and dementia, but the distinguishing characteristics are twofold: delirium manifests with an alteration in alertness or level of consciousness and with a reduced capacity for cognitive processing, both of which appear within a short time frame; most dementias are slower in onset, and cognitive decline usually takes place in the setting of clear sensorium (although Dementia with Lewy Bodies can be characterized by altered sensorium and prominent perceptual distortions, such as hallucinations).

35. C: Despite evidence of resolve and appropriate self-care in dealing with difficult ex-boyfriends, a pattern of involvement in abusive relationships may exist that bears examination and intervention.

36. B: There are no absolute rules about self-disclosure, accepting small gifts, or touch, because the diverse cultural backgrounds and sociocultural situations of clients may make an action appropriate in one situation but inappropriate in another. However, it is never appropriate to allow romantic feelings or thoughts to interfere with clinical care. In such cases, supervision should be sought, and the situation should be monitored closely; it may become necessary for the client to be referred to another practitioner.

37. C: Any member of the family who prepares meals should be educated about the potential tyramine reaction that can occur with the ingestion of aged cheeses, certain sausages and other fermented protein products, and some alcoholic beverages (beer and wine). The presence of these products in food may be masked during preparation; therefore, both the food preparer and the patient should be aware of the risk.

38. A: A number of adequately designed and controlled studies have demonstrated the efficacy of stimulant medications, BPT, BCM, and peer-focused behavioral interventions in recreational settings in both children and adults with ADHD.

39. B: MAO inhibitor antidepressants—such as phenelzine, tranylcypromine, and isocarboxazid—are reserved for use until at least 3 or 4 other antidepressant options have failed to be helpful, because of the risk of toxic interactions with dietary items and other medications. The MAO inhibitor selegiline, applied as a patch, may circumvent some of these issues and may be categorized as a third- or fourth-line treatment.

40. B: No evidence indicates that lithium levels worsen psoriasis at the high end of the therapeutic range or are associated with improvement in psoriatic lesions at the lower end of the therapeutic range; therefore, blood monitoring is not helpful for managing lithium-associated psoriasis.

41. A: The aim of supportive psychotherapy is to help the patient through a difficult period by strengthening, supporting, and highlighting the patient's already existing strengths and assets. The duration of both the sessions themselves and of the course of therapy may be brief. Techniques of psychoanalysis meant to foster free association or even to provoke anxiety and uncertainty, such as the therapist presenting a "blank screen," tend to undermine or diminish usual defense mechanisms rather than strengthen them, as is the goal of supportive psychotherapies.

42. D: Phototherapy works better by increasing the intensity of light exposure rather than by increasing its duration, appears to be most effective when administered in the morning, and can have positive effects with as little as 30-45 minutes of exposure per day. Blue-green light may be the most effective part of the visual spectrum for treating depression.

43. C: The courts now require that practitioners relate sufficient information about alternative treatments that may be advantageous to the patient, discuss the possible risks and benefits associated with them, and discuss the option of no treatment.

44. B: The principle of autonomy holds that adults have the ability and the right to make reasonable and responsible choices for themselves. An adult woman in an abusive relationship may request counseling and even shelter, but the health practitioner is not mandated to report the situation to any civil or criminal authority, independent of the patient's willingness or consent. Doing so without the patient's consent would be a violation of confidentiality.

45. D: Financial indiscretion is not considered a reason for involuntary commitment for mental illness in most jurisdictions.

46. A: Piaget's 4 stages of cognitive development are Sensorimotor (birth to 2 years), Preoperational (ages 2-6 years), Concrete Operations (ages 6-12 years), and Formal Operations (ages 12-15+ years); Kohlberg's levels of moral development are Preconventional (ages 4-10 years), Conventional (ages 10-13 years and into adulthood), and Postconventional (from adolescence onward); Peplau's stages of personality development are Infancy (learning to count on others), Toddlerhood (learning to delay satisfaction), Early Childhood (identifying oneself), and Late Childhood (developing skills in participation); and Mahler's theory of separation-individuation includes the Autistic Phase (birth to 1 month), the Symbiotic Phase (ages 1-5 months), and the Separation-Individuation Phase (ages 5-36 months).

47. B: PHI does not include the name of the patient's physician, because this is not information that "identifies the individual or with respect to which there is a reasonable basis to believe the information can be used to identify the individual" (U.S. Department of Health and Human Services, 2003).

48. C: Veracity is the duty to tell the truth and not intentionally deceive or mislead clients. Occasions when the truth would produce harm or interfere with the recovery process are rare. The principle of autonomy holds that the patient is presumed rational and responsible, retaining the right to determine their own destiny and to be fully informed about their condition. Withholding the truth would violate this principle as well. In this case, the nurse is attempting to act under the principles of nonmaleficence (to do no intentional harm to the client), beneficence (to benefit or promote the good of others), and justice (to treat all individuals, including the family, equally and fairly); however, the primary duty is to the patient.

49. D: The chief reason to obtain consultation is to determine a professional assessment of whether a patient's situation is beyond your experience or knowledge to handle properly. Another reason to obtain consultation would be to honor the patient's requests for a second opinion, which should generally be facilitated. Although a second opinion provides a sharing of medical-legal responsibility, this is not the primary reason to obtain such.

50. C: Analytical Precision is not concerned with statistics and instruments. It refers to the decision-making process by which researchers synthesize concrete data (words of the subjects) into an

abstract that clarifies the meaning and the importance of the study. The last of the 5 criteria is Heuristic Relevance – The researcher clarifies the significance of the study, its applicability to public health or community nursing, and its likely influence on future research.

Secret Key #1 - Time is Your Greatest Enemy

Pace Yourself

Wear a watch. At the beginning of the test, check the time (or start a chronometer on your watch to count the minutes), and check the time after every few questions to make sure you are "on schedule."

If you are forced to speed up, do it efficiently. Usually one or more answer choices can be eliminated without too much difficulty. Above all, don't panic. Don't speed up and just begin guessing at random choices. By pacing yourself, and continually monitoring your progress against your watch, you will always know exactly how far ahead or behind you are with your available time. If you find that you are one minute behind on the test, don't skip one question without spending any time on it, just to catch back up. Take 15 fewer seconds on the next four questions, and after four questions you'll have caught back up. Once you catch back up, you can continue working each problem at your normal pace.

Furthermore, don't dwell on the problems that you were rushed on. If a problem was taking up too much time and you made a hurried guess, it must be difficult. The difficult questions are the ones you are most likely to miss anyway, so it isn't a big loss. It is better to end with more time than you need than to run out of time.

Lastly, sometimes it is beneficial to slow down if you are constantly getting ahead of time. You are always more likely to catch a careless mistake by working more slowly than quickly, and among very high-scoring test takers (those who are likely to have lots of time left over), careless errors affect the score more than mastery of material.

Secret Key #2 - Guessing is not Guesswork

You probably know that guessing is a good idea. Unlike other standardized tests, there is no penalty for getting a wrong answer. Even if you have no idea about a question, you still have a 20-25% chance of getting it right.

Most test takers do not understand the impact that proper guessing can have on their score. Unless you score extremely high, guessing will significantly contribute to your final score.

Monkeys Take the Test

What most test takers don't realize is that to insure that 20-25% chance, you have to guess randomly. If you put 20 monkeys in a room to take this test, assuming they answered once per question and behaved themselves, on average they would get 20-25% of the questions correct. Put 20 test takers in the room, and the average will be much lower among guessed questions. Why?

1. The test writers intentionally write deceptive answer choices that "look" right. A test taker has no idea about a question, so he picks the "best looking" answer, which is often wrong. The monkey has no idea what looks good and what doesn't, so it will consistently be right about 20-25% of the time.

2. Test takers will eliminate answer choices from the guessing pool based on a hunch or intuition. Simple but correct answers often get excluded, leaving a 0% chance of being correct. The monkey has no clue, and often gets lucky with the best choice.

This is why the process of elimination endorsed by most test courses is flawed and detrimental to your performance. Test takers don't guess; they make an ignorant stab in the dark that is usually worse than random.

$5 Challenge

Let me introduce one of the most valuable ideas of this course—the $5 challenge:

You only mark your "best guess" if you are willing to bet $5 on it.
You only eliminate choices from guessing if you are willing to bet $5 on it.

Why $5? Five dollars is an amount of money that is small yet not insignificant, and can really add up fast (20 questions could cost you $100). Likewise, each answer choice on one question of the test will have a small impact on your overall score, but it can really add up to a lot of points in the end.

The process of elimination IS valuable. The following shows your chance of guessing it right:

If you eliminate wrong answer choices until only this many remain:	Chance of getting it correct:
1	100%
2	50%
3	33%

However, if you accidentally eliminate the right answer or go on a hunch for an incorrect answer, your chances drop dramatically—to 0%. By guessing among all the answer choices, you are GUARANTEED to have a shot at the right answer.

That's why the $5 test is so valuable. If you give up the advantage and safety of a pure guess, it had better be worth the risk.

What we still haven't covered is how to be sure that whatever guess you make is truly random. Here's the easiest way:

Always pick the first answer choice among those remaining.

Such a technique means that you have decided, **before you see a single test question**, exactly how you are going to guess, and since the order of choices tells you nothing about which one is correct, this guessing technique is perfectly random.

This section is not meant to scare you away from making educated guesses or eliminating choices; you just need to define when a choice is worth eliminating. The $5 test, along with a pre-defined random guessing strategy, is the best way to make sure you reap all of the benefits of guessing.

Secret Key #3 - Practice Smarter, Not Harder

Many test takers delay the test preparation process because they dread the awful amounts of practice time they think necessary to succeed on the test. We have refined an effective method that will take you only a fraction of the time.

There are a number of "obstacles" in the path to success. Among these are answering questions, finishing in time, and mastering test-taking strategies. All must be executed on the day of the test at peak performance, or your score will suffer. The test is a mental marathon that has a large impact on your future.

Just like a marathon runner, it is important to work your way up to the full challenge. So first you just worry about questions, and then time, and finally strategy:

Success Strategy

1. Find a good source for practice tests.
2. If you are willing to make a larger time investment, consider using more than one study guide. Often the different approaches of multiple authors will help you "get" difficult concepts.
3. Take a practice test with no time constraints, with all study helps, "open book." Take your time with questions and focus on applying strategies.
4. Take a practice test with time constraints, with all guides, "open book."
5. Take a final practice test without open material and with time limits.

If you have time to take more practice tests, just repeat step 5. By gradually exposing yourself to the full rigors of the test environment, you will condition your mind to the stress of test day and maximize your success.

Secret Key #4 - Prepare, Don't Procrastinate

Let me state an obvious fact: if you take the test three times, you will probably get three different scores. This is due to the way you feel on test day, the level of preparedness you have, and the version of the test you see. Despite the test writers' claims to the contrary, some versions of the test WILL be easier for you than others.

Since your future depends so much on your score, you should maximize your chances of success. In order to maximize the likelihood of success, you've got to prepare in advance. This means taking practice tests and spending time learning the information and test taking strategies you will need to succeed.

Never go take the actual test as a "practice" test, expecting that you can just take it again if you need to. Take all the practice tests you can on your own, but when you go to take the official test, be prepared, be focused, and do your best the first time!

Secret Key #5 - Test Yourself

Everyone knows that time is money. There is no need to spend too much of your time or too little of your time preparing for the test. You should only spend as much of your precious time preparing as is necessary for you to get the score you need.

Once you have taken a practice test under real conditions of time constraints, then you will know if you are ready for the test or not.

If you have scored extremely high the first time that you take the practice test, then there is not much point in spending countless hours studying. You are already there.

Benchmark your abilities by retaking practice tests and seeing how much you have improved. Once you consistently score high enough to guarantee success, then you are ready.

If you have scored well below where you need, then knuckle down and begin studying in earnest. Check your improvement regularly through the use of practice tests under real conditions. Above all, don't worry, panic, or give up. The key is perseverance!

Then, when you go to take the test, remain confident and remember how well you did on the practice tests. If you can score high enough on a practice test, then you can do the same on the real thing.

General Strategies

The most important thing you can do is to ignore your fears and jump into the test immediately. Do not be overwhelmed by any strange-sounding terms. You have to jump into the test like jumping into a pool—all at once is the easiest way.

Make Predictions

As you read and understand the question, try to guess what the answer will be. Remember that several of the answer choices are wrong, and once you begin reading them, your mind will immediately become cluttered with answer choices designed to throw you off. Your mind is typically the most focused immediately after you have read the question and digested its contents. If you can, try to predict what the correct answer will be. You may be surprised at what you can predict.

Quickly scan the choices and see if your prediction is in the listed answer choices. If it is, then you can be quite confident that you have the right answer. It still won't hurt to check the other answer choices, but most of the time, you've got it!

Answer the Question

It may seem obvious to only pick answer choices that answer the question, but the test writers can create some excellent answer choices that are wrong. Don't pick an answer just because it sounds right, or you believe it to be true. It MUST answer the question. Once you've made your selection, always go back and check it against the question and make sure that you didn't misread the question and that the answer choice does answer the question posed.

Benchmark

After you read the first answer choice, decide if you think it sounds correct or not. If it doesn't, move on to the next answer choice. If it does, mentally mark that answer choice. This doesn't mean that you've definitely selected it as your answer choice, it just means that it's the best you've seen thus far. Go ahead and read the next choice. If the next choice is worse than the one you've already selected, keep going to the next answer choice. If the next choice is better than the choice you've already selected, mentally mark the new answer choice as your best guess.

The first answer choice that you select becomes your standard. Every other answer choice must be benchmarked against that standard. That choice is correct until proven otherwise by another answer choice beating it out. Once you've decided that no other answer choice seems as good, do one final check to ensure that your answer choice answers the question posed.

Valid Information

Don't discount any of the information provided in the question. Every piece of information may be necessary to determine the correct answer. None of the information in the question is there to throw you off (while the answer choices will certainly have information to throw you off). If two seemingly unrelated topics are discussed, don't ignore either. You can be confident there is a relationship, or it wouldn't be included in the question, and you are probably going to have to determine what is that relationship to find the answer.

Avoid "Fact Traps"

Don't get distracted by a choice that is factually true. Your search is for the answer that answers the question. Stay focused and don't fall for an answer that is true but irrelevant. Always go back to the question and make sure you're choosing an answer that actually answers the question and is not just a true statement. An answer can be factually correct, but it MUST answer the question asked. Additionally, two answers can both be seemingly correct, so be sure to read all of the answer choices, and make sure that you get the one that BEST answers the question.

Milk the Question

Some of the questions may throw you completely off. They might deal with a subject you have not been exposed to, or one that you haven't reviewed in years. While your lack of knowledge about the subject will be a hindrance, the question itself can give you many clues that will help you find the correct answer. Read the question carefully and look for clues. Watch particularly for adjectives and nouns describing difficult terms or words that you don't recognize. Regardless of whether you completely understand a word or not, replacing it with a synonym, either provided or one you more familiar with, may help you to understand what the questions are asking. Rather than wracking your mind about specific detailed information concerning a difficult term or word, try to use mental substitutes that are easier to understand.

The Trap of Familiarity

Don't just choose a word because you recognize it. On difficult questions, you may not recognize a number of words in the answer choices. The test writers don't put "make-believe" words on the test, so don't think that just because you only recognize all the words in one answer choice that that answer choice must be correct. If you only recognize words in one answer choice, then focus on that one. Is it correct? Try your best to determine if it is correct. If it is, that's great. If not, eliminate it. Each word and answer choice you eliminate increases your chances of getting the question correct, even if you then have to guess among the unfamiliar choices.

Eliminate Answers

Eliminate choices as soon as you realize they are wrong. But be careful! Make sure you consider all of the possible answer choices. Just because one appears right, doesn't mean that the next one won't be even better! The test writers will usually put more than one good answer choice for every question, so read all of them. Don't worry if you are stuck between two that seem right. By getting down to just two remaining possible choices, your odds are now 50/50. Rather than wasting too much time, play the odds. You are guessing, but guessing wisely because you've been able to knock out some of the answer choices that you know are wrong. If you are eliminating choices and realize that the last answer choice you are left with is also obviously wrong, don't panic. Start over and consider each choice again. There may easily be something that you missed the first time and will realize on the second pass.

Tough Questions

If you are stumped on a problem or it appears too hard or too difficult, don't waste time. Move on! Remember though, if you can quickly check for obviously incorrect answer choices, your chances of guessing correctly are greatly improved. Before you completely give up, at least try to knock out a couple of possible answers. Eliminate what you can and then guess at the remaining answer choices before moving on.

Brainstorm

If you get stuck on a difficult question, spend a few seconds quickly brainstorming. Run through the complete list of possible answer choices. Look at each choice and ask yourself, "Could this answer the question satisfactorily?" Go through each answer choice and consider it independently of the others. By systematically going through all possibilities, you may find something that you would otherwise overlook. Remember though that when you get stuck, it's important to try to keep moving.

Read Carefully

Understand the problem. Read the question and answer choices carefully. Don't miss the question because you misread the terms. You have plenty of time to read each question thoroughly and make sure you understand what is being asked. Yet a happy medium must be attained, so don't waste too much time. You must read carefully, but efficiently.

Face Value

When in doubt, use common sense. Always accept the situation in the problem at face value. Don't read too much into it. These problems will not require you to make huge leaps of logic. The test writers aren't trying to throw you off with a cheap trick. If you have to go beyond creativity and make a leap of logic in order to have an answer choice answer the question, then you should look at the other answer choices. Don't overcomplicate the problem by creating theoretical relationships or explanations that will warp time or space. These are normal problems rooted in reality. It's just that the applicable relationship or explanation may not be readily apparent and you have to figure things out. Use your common sense to interpret anything that isn't clear.

Prefixes

If you're having trouble with a word in the question or answer choices, try dissecting it. Take advantage of every clue that the word might include. Prefixes and suffixes can be a huge help. Usually they allow you to determine a basic meaning. Pre- means before, post- means after, pro - is positive, de- is negative. From these prefixes and suffixes, you can get an idea of the general meaning of the word and try to put it into context. Beware though of any traps. Just because con- is the opposite of pro-, doesn't necessarily mean congress is the opposite of progress!

Hedge Phrases

Watch out for critical hedge phrases, led off with words such as "likely," "may," "can," "sometimes," "often," "almost," "mostly," "usually," "generally," "rarely," and "sometimes." Question writers insert these hedge phrases to cover every possibility. Often an answer choice will be wrong simply because it leaves no room for exception. Unless the situation calls for them, avoid answer choices that have definitive words like "exactly," and "always."

Switchback Words

Stay alert for "switchbacks." These are the words and phrases frequently used to alert you to shifts in thought. The most common switchback word is "but." Others include "although," "however," "nevertheless," "on the other hand," "even though," "while," "in spite of," "despite," and "regardless of."

New Information

Correct answer choices will rarely have completely new information included. Answer choices typically are straightforward reflections of the material asked about and will directly relate to the question. If a new piece of information is included in an answer choice that doesn't even seem to relate to the topic being asked about, then that answer choice is likely incorrect. All of the information needed to answer the question is usually provided for you in the question. You should not have to make guesses that are unsupported or choose answer choices that require unknown information that cannot be reasoned from what is given.

Time Management

On technical questions, don't get lost on the technical terms. Don't spend too much time on any one question. If you don't know what a term means, then odds are you aren't going to get much further since you don't have a dictionary. You should be able to immediately recognize whether or not you know a term. If you don't, work with the other clues that you have—the other answer choices and terms provided—but don't waste too much time trying to figure out a difficult term that you don't know.

Contextual Clues

Look for contextual clues. An answer can be right but not the correct answer. The contextual clues will help you find the answer that is most right and is correct. Understand the context in which a phrase or statement is made. This will help you make important distinctions.

Don't Panic

Panicking will not answer any questions for you; therefore, it isn't helpful. When you first see the question, if your mind goes blank, take a deep breath. Force yourself to mechanically go through the steps of solving the problem using the strategies you've learned.

Pace Yourself

Don't get clock fever. It's easy to be overwhelmed when you're looking at a page full of questions, your mind is full of random thoughts and feeling confused, and the clock is ticking down faster than you would like. Calm down and maintain the pace that you have set for yourself. As long as you are on track by monitoring your pace, you are guaranteed to have enough time for yourself. When you get to the last few minutes of the test, it may seem like you won't have enough time left, but if you only have as many questions as you should have left at that point, then you're right on track!

Answer Selection

The best way to pick an answer choice is to eliminate all of those that are wrong, until only one is left and confirm that is the correct answer. Sometimes though, an answer choice may immediately look right. Be careful! Take a second to make sure that the other choices are not equally obvious. Don't make a hasty mistake. There are only two times that you should stop before checking other answers. First is when you are positive that the answer choice you have selected is correct. Second is when time is almost out and you have to make a quick guess!

Check Your Work

Since you will probably not know every term listed and the answer to every question, it is important that you get credit for the ones that you do know. Don't miss any questions through careless mistakes. If at all possible, try to take a second to look back over your answer selection and make sure you've selected the correct answer choice and haven't made a costly careless mistake (such as marking an answer choice that you didn't mean to mark). The time it takes for this quick double check should more than pay for itself in caught mistakes.

Beware of Directly Quoted Answers

Sometimes an answer choice will repeat word for word a portion of the question or reference section. However, beware of such exact duplication. It may be a trap! More than likely, the correct choice will paraphrase or summarize a point, rather than being exactly the same wording.

Slang

Scientific sounding answers are better than slang ones. An answer choice that begins "To compare the outcomes..." is much more likely to be correct than one that begins "Because some people insisted..."

Extreme Statements

Avoid wild answers that throw out highly controversial ideas that are proclaimed as established fact. An answer choice that states the "process should used in certain situations, if..." is much more likely to be correct than one that states the "process should be discontinued completely." The first is a calm rational statement and doesn't even make a definitive, uncompromising stance, using a hedge word "if" to provide wiggle room, whereas the second choice is a radical idea and far more extreme.

Answer Choice Families

When you have two or more answer choices that are direct opposites or parallels, one of them is usually the correct answer. For instance, if one answer choice states "x increases" and another answer choice states "x decreases" or "y increases," then those two or three answer choices are very similar in construction and fall into the same family of answer choices. A family of answer choices consists of two or three answer choices, very similar in construction, but often with directly opposite meanings. Usually the correct answer choice will be in that family of answer choices. The "odd man out" or answer choice that doesn't seem to fit the parallel construction of the other answer choices is more likely to be incorrect.